One Third of Your Stomach

One Third of Your Stomach

The food and
lifestyle philosophy
that draws you
closer to God

JULIDE TURKER-GULER

Note: All Qur'an references used in this book come from
The Qur'an: A Translation for the 21st Century, translated by Adil Salahi.
Salahi, A 2019, *The Qur'an: A Translation for the 21st Century,* The
Islamic Foundation, Markfield, Leicestershire, United Kingdom.

First pub ished in 2023 by Dean Publishing
PO Box 119
Mt. Macedon, Victoria, 3441
Australia
deanpublishing.com

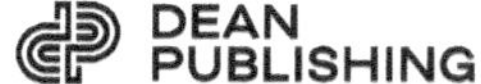

Cataloguing-in-Publication Data
National Library of Australia
Title: One Third of Your Stomach
Edition: 1st edn
ISBN: 978-1-925452-59-4
Category: Nutrition/Herbal Medicine/Islamic practices

DEDICATION

To my mother, my mother, my mother, and then my father.

CONTENTS

PART ONE
The Mind, Body, and Spirit Connection

PART TWO
The Intersection of Food and Faith

TERMS AND DEFINITIONS

Ayah: omen, sign, proof, commandment.

Caliphate: chief Muslim ruler.

Fitrah: original disposition/natural constitution.

Hadith: a collection of traditions and proverbs of the Prophet, Muhammad (peace be upon him).

Halal: method for preparing meat as prescribed by Muslim law.

Haq: Arabic word for truth, and, in Islamic context, it is interpreted as 'right' or 'reality'.

Madrasah: Arabic word for a college for Islamic instruction.

Nafs: translated as meaning 'self' and also referenced as 'ego', 'soul', 'psyche'.

PBUH: said every time the Prophet is mentioned as a show of respect and is an acronym for 'peace be upon Him'.

SAW: means PBUH in Arabic.

Sharia law: based on Islamic scriptures, Sharia is Islam's body of law.

Sunna: Sunna, also spelled Sunnah, are the traditions and practices of the Islamic prophet, Muhammad, that constitute a model for Muslims to follow. The Sunna are what all the Muslims of Muhammad's time evidently saw, followed, and passed on to the next generations.

Surah: a chapter of the Qur'an.

Tayyib: good, pleasant, something that is lawful, permissible.

Tasbih: Arabic word for prayer beads used as counting aid in reciting titles of God's names, and so on, in meditation.

Vicegerent: a person regarded as an earthly representative of God.

Wudu: in Arabic means ablution, in English – a set of physical purification steps for Muslims to do before they pray.

INTRODUCTION

As humans, we have a level of consciousness above all that has been created by the Divine. We have an ability to differentiate right from wrong, and we have an intellect above everything else that has been created. We also possess the power of choice, and it alone creates a clear-cut vision of why God has declared humans as the vicegerents of all other creation.

So, it is no surprise that logic tells us we can understand the importance of health and wellness and its influence on our overall lives. We have the capacity to acknowledge animal ethics; we have a spiritual component to our three-dimensional bodies, and we have an ability to consciously live. The way to live our fullest lives goes hand in hand with our divine reason for being on this earth plane, serving our creator through living consciously.

The concept of keeping our physical and spiritual vessel 'clean', so to speak, is the core philosophy of our religion. It is in the Qur'an and in the practice of our prophet, Muhammad's (PBUH), life.

Self-care is about treating your physical and emotional body with deep-rooted respect, through honouring its processes and giving it its due right. Its due right is beautifully and coherently outlined through the Qur'an and through the Sunna (teachings and practices of Muhammad, peace be upon him). This is because the body is given to us in trust: it does not belong to us, per se. It belongs to God, and it is to be returned to God. As a matter of fact, the Qur'an promises that "every soul shall taste death" (21:35). For believers of the Islamic faith, this is a transition of our spiritual body from a three-dimensional world to a four-dimensional universe, where the body is not required; thus, it is left on this plane. Our bodies are just physical vessels in which we manifest our spiritual selves; hence, its wellness determines the wellness of our spiritual and emotional selves.

Self-care, to many, as I have observed in daily conversations and on social media, is limited to getting our nails done, having a spa pamper session, or having a massage. It is limited to practices that more so morph the visual of the physical body. However, this is not the type of self-care I am referring to. Self-care is not limited to getting a massage after a long week with the kids or having a coffee with friends. You may suggest that these are versions of self-care, but they are very superficial in their nature, unable to satiate the spiritual void but capable of satiating the sense of ego.

The true essence of self-care lies within the foundations of self-compassion and, as a result, respect for our physical and emotional bodies that carry out their jobs on the physical earth plane. It embodies the fact that the body is temporarily given to man in trust to fulfil the objectives of this three-dimensional experience. In order to create a meaningful life, serving the purpose of creation, self-care must be ingrained in everything that makes the physical vessel stay clean and, therefore, work efficiently and effectively and, as a result, serve its purpose to its fullest.

This concept of self-care includes what we eat, what we drink, and the very essence of how the food gets to our plates, including the importance of ethical farming practices, the treatment of animals with dignity, whether the vegetables were sprayed with poisons that alter their ability to produce nutrients, among many other considerations.

Self-care also encompasses the people involved in the farms and factories, those who help in the production and supply of food. Are they treated well? Are they paid well? Do they have, at minimum, their basic human rights and needs met? It is important to acknowledge whether chemicals, packaging, or processing has affected and interfered with the very flow of the food's divine energy. Will the food serve me in being a connection, an energy channel to the Divine? Will it provide me with the mental and physical power to serve my Lord in this physical vessel? Or will it draw me away from him?

Self-care is understanding that we eat to live; we do not live to eat. Food serves a purpose outside of leisurely gluttony, which is a purpose we have given it in this day and age. The Prophet, when he passed away (PBUH), was observed to have no extra weight, no belly fat, because he never ate more than his fill.

An overweight man was once told that had he eaten less, one other hungry person could have been satiated with the excess food he had consumed. But we don't just eat because we are gluttonous in nature – not at all. We eat because we have an emotional need to connect with food, a problem many of us experience, as we turn to food for comfort. We have a biochemical desire to connect with food because it increases brain chemicals called neurotransmitters, such as serotonin and GABA, that make us feel happy. It gives us an instant relief from any pain and suffering, an instant distraction, however short-lived it may be.

Let Us Take a Journey Together

Throughout this book, we will explore important questions and unearth critical answers that help us better understand our religion, how to better apply it to our lives, and how to best serve the Creator through conscious living, hence, fulfilling our reason for creation. Together, we will not only explore and learn the physical 'rules and regulations' around food consumption from an Islamic perspective, but we will also gain a thorough understanding of the overall philosophy. Because with understanding comes a genuine ability to apply the learning, to transfer the energy of knowledge into action – and we know that knowledge is incomplete unless it is married to action.

The companions of our beloved Prophet Muhammad (PBUH) would go to him for advice and rulings around matters. They would apply this advice to their lives, and they would only come back for the next piece of wisdom once the one before had become a lifestyle, which generally took months.

We are in the age of excess information, where we 'know' because information is freely available. But most of what we know, we do not understand. Sometimes we do understand; however, the information is conflicting. Sometimes it comes to us in the form of oppression and tyranny, so we complacently comply because we have trauma associated with people pleasing and not being able to create space for ourselves as we pass this life in our own shadow, unaware of our potential, too scared to take up space.

Therefore, I pray wholeheartedly that this book empowers you to hold light to your strengths and enables you to work on your weaknesses. I pray it either makes your convictions or breaks them but, either way, allows you to stand strong and independent in your own light, your own sense of self-worth, your own intuition, which I always accept as a connection to the divine. I pray that we strive to do our level best to apply the teachings in this book, one step at a time, acknowledging that it is okay, no matter where we are in our journey, that there are things we can learn. I pray that we come from a place of compassion for ourselves, being okay with the fact that a lot of unlearning and relearning will be involved. We will create space for the mental and physical metamorphosis without comparing ourselves to another, and we will wholeheartedly understand that this is a part of the growth process, a part of the process of gaining wisdom, clarity, and centredness. This is a gentle nudge to help recalibrate ourselves and reconnect us with the powers within and external to us.

My job through this book is to inspire you to find the light, the wisdom, the motivation to make changes, one step at a time. Through doing right comes a sense of satisfaction and contentment, a sense of connectedness with our purpose of creation, which is the only right way I know to fill the void that we, at times, feel in our hearts. As we journey through our short-lived time on this earth plane, there will be many fads that encourage us to fill our voids with them: the next fad gadget or fashion item, the next fad diet, the next fad self-care regimen, the next fad get-rich-quick scheme, and so on, and so forth. But none of these things grant us true spiritual fulfilment.

Our Responsibility

Islam leaves nothing to ambiguity. When we connect to our manual, the Qur'an, and read it in the light of our prophetic teachings, our understanding allows us to convert the information into action with ease. The logic and simplicity of the Islamic way of food consumption, for example, is rather straightforward. You don't need to be a Muslim to be a conscious consumer, and every conscious consumer is not, in fact, a Muslim. Simple, logical connections with our Earth, such as eating in season, preventing overconsumption, eating one third of our stomach's volume, getting ample exercise through regular daily activities, and waiting for the previous meal to digest before consuming the next are the basic core fundamentals of the 1400-year-old food and lifestyle philosophy that is gifted to us in the Qur'an by the best of man, Muhammad (PBUH).

It includes values that honour others and other creatures, such as ensuring we are not stomping over the rights of those in the plant and animal kingdoms, with whom we share this planet. As Allah has blessed us with the ability to think, and with intelligence and intellect, it has become our duty of care to look out for those whose rights are left to our discretion, such as animals and our environment. "Are those who know equal to those who do not know? Only they will remember [who are] people of understanding" (Qur'an 39:9).

This gentle religion of ours only holds us accountable for what we know; it does not hold us accountable for what we do not know. It does, however, hold us accountable and responsible for seeking knowledge. When there is no awareness, there is no responsibility. However, developing the awareness requires knowledge, and we are responsible for seeking that knowledge.

Together, we will learn the important role that a healthy body and a healthy mind has in helping us connect with our higher selves and responding to the calls of serving our creator through conscious living. We will explore lifestyle habits that our prophet implemented and how these very actions align with current science and medicine – a womb to tomb philosophy to help us become the level best versions of ourselves, emotionally, spiritually, and physically.

You may be asking, "What about those of us who have tried all of the above but are still emotionally unwell?" Or, "Is sickness not a test from God? Doesn't the Qur'an say we will be tested with our health and our wealth, like those who were tested before us? Isn't everything in the control of God?"

Let me answer. As people of intellect, we do not sit in the back seat of this car called life. We know that what we have no control over is when we are born and when we die. Outside of that, we have some level of conscious, intellectual, financial, and social control over our lives. The line that separates the concepts of destiny and free will can sometimes look blurry. As people of consciousness and intellect, we have an ability to make choices in many aspects of our lives.

Let me give you an example. There are many people we know, which may include ourselves as the very readers of this book, who smoke, who drink, who eat very poor diets, who live very sedentary lifestyles; however, there seems to be 'not much' wrong with them from a health perspective, for now. Then there are those who eat well, exercise, and do all the meditation and spirituality work but suffer significant health challenges. Oftentimes, we chose to give examples of situations that don't really happen that often. Potentially, it may be a means of silencing a guilty subconscious mind. Essentially, we are trying hard to justify the choices we make. We try to convince ourselves that, whether we choose to make a difference in those mentioned areas or not, whatever will happen will happen. Que sera, sera – whatever will be, will be.

Does that mean we are void of conscious responsibility? And if we are completely void of responsibility, how come we are created as men of intellect and choice and not as angels, whose sole purpose is to serve God? We *do* have choice and responsibility, which means we are not void of the outcomes; instead, we are wholly responsible for them. God says in the Qur'an (4:79), "Whatever good happens to you is from Allah; and whatever misfortune smites you is because of your own action." So, in essence, we like to take outlier examples of anecdotal experiences in life to fit our own agendas, as opposed to accepting the truth for what it is.

The person who took care of their body as best as possible and still experienced a debilitating disease was certainly undergoing a test from God. They did their level best to prevent disease but were still tested with it. When, on the other hand, someone does nothing to better their physical self and disease strikes them, they created the reason; they planted the seeds and must reap what grows.

Fixing Our Spiritual Compass

In my opinion, and in the opinion of highly reputable Islamic scholars, most modern diseases are lifestyle- and diet-related. Potentially, this is the case because we have lost the calibre of our spiritual compass and, instead, have focused primarily on the physical compass. What does this mean? For the most part, we have only kept consistent with the physical requirements of Islam, such as praying, covering up, fasting, and going to hajj. But we have disconnected from the important requirements, which feed the spiritual body, such as zikr (a form of Islamic meditation or invocation), applying empathy and leading by example as Muhammad (PBUH) did, approaching every situation with empathy and kindness, spreading love, forgiving, holding space for another, feeding our bodies only what they need and not a morsel more, focusing on food being a means of keeping our backs straight, eating our fill to live, not living to eat, and so on, and so forth.

Much of the time, we remain victims of the very same circumstances we create for ourselves; hence, the stories we cherrypick are often to mask our own shortcomings, mostly because we do not necessarily have the capacity or the tools and resources to know what to do with the emotions that otherwise come up and haunt us. They are parts of us that we continue to hide in our own shadows. We fail to live lives of true knowledge seeking, true humbleness, and true vulnerability, which comprise our essence as humans.

The point is, if we genuinely eat well, exercise, and do all those things that we know are good for us, and we develop a health condition, then we are not to blame, right? We have done our absolute best on every single level; however, Allah has chosen to give us the gift of illness. We put our trust in Allah and say the illness is from him, as a test. After all, we know the verse in the Qur'an and find ourselves quoting it often: "Do the people think that they will be left to say, 'We believe' and they will not be tried? But We have certainly tried those before them, and Allah will surely make evident those who are truthful, and He will surely make evident the liars" (29:2–3).

On the other hand, there are those of us who create the right conditions for diseases to develop via neglecting our health, sometimes to such an extent that we don't only allow for disease to thrive, but we also jeopardise our potential to heal.

This self-sabotage may genuinely occur because we don't yet understand the impact it is having on us on a wider scale. Or perhaps it is an unconscious effort to punish ourselves. It isn't just the calories that count; it is also the damage that is being done to the body as a whole. On a cellular level, this is not just creating opportunity for cancers and the like, but it is also creating opportunities for disconnecting from our core purpose, disconnecting from our ability to serve our creator, causing us to 'lose' time via trying to mend the health lost, causing us to lose the ability to connect with our higher selves, which is, in essence, the very core purpose of our creation as believers.

How Connected Are We?

The next time you say, "I have raised my kids like this, and they are fine" or, "I have been eating this way, and I am fine," remember to elaborate on what fine means, as fine is a relative term. Get curious with yourself and with your kids. How connected are our children with God? And how connected are they with themselves?

Often, when consulting children or adults, I ask the questions:

- ✧ "Are you opening your bowels daily?"
- ✧ "How is your memory?"
- ✧ "What did you eat yesterday?"

Much of the time, to my despair, the answers don't come very easily at all. Why? Because we generally pass through life on autopilot, with a lack of presence. Get curious about how food affects your lifestyle habits, such as not being able to wake up for morning prayer or not being able to keep your ablution (the physical cleansing steps required prior to prayer), or even how this translates to our behaviour towards others in our homes. Get curious about whether you fully understand everything you read or whether you read the same sentence over and over again and don't understand the essence of it.

Many of us feel anxious about the idea of sitting with our own thoughts; thus, we constantly distract ourselves with being busy to the extent that we take the phone into the toilet with us. Sometimes, we are aware that this is just a means to keep our minds distracted from the otherwise uncomfortable feelings that will come to play, but we continue the behaviour anyway.

Most of us come from families whose parents and grandparents come from a generation of immigrants. Since the Great Depression, we have decreased our expectations for the human mind and body, limiting ourselves to having shelter, food, and safety because, back then, we were robbed of those basic human rights and needs. Although these things are very important, in the safety and security we currently live in, we can now reconnect with other spiritual and physical needs to consciously serve humanity.

When we are physically unwell, it leads to a plethora of issues with trying to fulfil our Islamic obligations, such as being unable to pray wholeheartedly due to the fatigue we are experiencing, or we cannot hold our ablution due to having an unhealthy digestive system. It can also cause other issues, such as losing patience, lacking tolerance with others, and not being able to empathise with others, all contributing to a poor-quality lifestyle.

When we have low vibrational energy, we attract everything on the same frequency and instead of sujood (aka child's pose for those of you who are familiar with yoga) lifting the world off our shoulders, it puts the world's weight onto our shoulders.

Therefore... IQRA... `iqra bismi rabbika lladhee khalaqa 2 khalaqa l-insaana min `alaqin 3 iqra wa rabbuka l-akramu 4 alladhee `allama bil-qalami 5 `allama l-insaana ma lam ya`lam.

"Let us recite in the name of our lord, who created man from a clinging substance. Let us recite... and our lord is most generous, who taught by the pen, taught man that which he knew not..." (Qur'an 96:1–6).

PART ONE

The Mind, Body, and Spirit Connection

CHAPTER ONE

INTRODUCTION TO PROPHETIC MEDICINE (*ṬIBB AN-NABAWĪ*)

God creates man and says,
"Mankind is the vicegerent, he is the custodian
on earth." It is a man's job to protect everything
that is a part of nature – from the insects to
the birds, from the trees to the animals.

Every Muslim is the recipient, guardian, and executor of God's will on Earth; his responsibilities are all encompassing. A Muslim's duty to act in defence of what is right is as much part of his faith as is his duty to oppose wrong. The Prophet (PBUH) once said, "If someone among you sees wrong, he must right it by his hand if he can (deed, conduct, action). If he cannot, then by his tongue (speak up, verbally oppose); if he cannot, then by his gaze (silent expression of disapproval); and if he cannot, then in his heart. The last is the minimum expression of his conviction (faith, courage)".[1]

Principles of Prophetic Medicine

Traditionally in Islam, there is a guide for all facets of life, from wider concepts of faith and morality to the practicalities of daily living. We are directed as to how we should treat others and ourselves, how often and in what manner we should pray, what we should eat, when we should fast, and how our dead should be buried. We are taught to decipher right from wrong, good from evil, and desire from need.

Of the many aspects of life in which Islam proffers guidance, there are two that I will be focusing on in this book. The first is the preservation of health, and the other is treatment of disease.

Our prophet, Muhammad (PBUH), was the epitome of what the vicegerent is supposed to be. He was put on this earth to guide people – as model and teacher – in all aspects of life, including health. So, a collection of his sayings and actions were compiled, and this is what guided, and continues to guide, his followers. Prophet Muhammad's (PBUH) principles that refer to health, we collectively accept as being prophetic medicine – *Tibb Al-Nabawi* in Arabic.

When we look at health from a prophetic medicine perspective, we are guided as to how to maintain our wellbeing and if we are to be sick, how to treat that illness. Prophetic medicine is not just about eating particular foods or focusing on how you physically feel; it is a way of life. It is about how you feed your mind and your spirit, as well as the physical vessel.

When preventing or treating disease, prophetic medicine considers the whole individual rather than just a body part or organ in isolation. This is in direct contrast to modern medicine, which treats illness using a linear paradigm. One of the biggest challenges of conventional medicine is that as long as we disconnect the human from its environment and spiritual self, we will always fail. We are interconnected with nature and with the divine realm. To discount those facets of human experience means we cannot achieve optimum health. We talk more about this in chapter two.

Background of Sickness and Wellness in Islamic and Pre-Islamic Arabia

Pagan Arabia (Arabia before Islam) consisted primarily of the area now known as Saudi Arabia and existed prior to the seventh century CE.[2] It was a world filled with endemic diseases, such as tuberculosis, rickets, scurvy, leprosy, malaria, and gastrointestinal illness.[3]

Due to poor climate conditions, social injustice, poverty, and ignorance, the level of health was very low. The soil was fertile for disease – there was a lack of clean water, and the nutritional status was poor.[4] Many people lived in poverty, so they did not have access to fresh produce, even if it was growing in season. Due to this shortage of food, the people lived off a monotonous diet that did not provide a high level of nourishment. Part of the issue was the absence of conscious knowledge regarding the importance of what we are and how that translated into good mental and physical health. Medicine was folkloric, where surgical knowledge was limited to primitive cauterisation (a practice where the body is burnt to seal a wound or remove a part of it) and branding, which were very harsh forms of treatment.[5]

In the time of the pharaohs, human sacrifice was customary. Child infanticide was common, and newborn females were prone to premature death. Daughters were sometimes buried alive to avoid poverty or shame.[6] Women were seen as a commodity, and some practices involved a man throwing something on a woman to claim her as his property if her husband had died. The belief system that drove countries like Saudi Arabia was paganism, which involved the worship of multiple gods through statues or idols. These deities delighted in sensual pleasures and material goods. Much of the belief system was set around natural cycles of birth, growth, and death, absent of any teachings of Moses, Jesus, Abraham or any other prophet who had walked the Earth pre-Muhammad.

As a result, a lot of emotional trauma was inflicted upon the community. This oppression and the stress of daily life meant that alcohol became a psychological necessity for pre-Islamic Arabs to cope. Initially, the Bedouins of Arabia had no knowledge of wine until the migrant Christians arrived and gifted it to their newly converted Christian brothers. Thus, a culture of intoxication did not take long to spread rampantly as drinking became a habit, especially due to the lack of alcohol prohibition in the pagan belief system.[7]

Muhammad (PBUH) grew up in this context, but he was not a Christian nor a pagan. He worked as a merchant and was considered a trustworthy man, earning the nickname, 'Al Amin', which means 'the trustworthy'. Muhammad was spiritually aligned with the natural cycle of the world and known for his kindness, trust, and compassion.

As he grew older, he began meditating for long periods of time, seeking solitude within a cave at Mount Hira, just north of Mecca. In 609 CE, at age 40, he was visited by the angel, Gabriel, and received the first revelation from God. According to the Islamic philosophy, this is known as the Night of Power (*Laylat al-Qadr*).

Gabriel told Muhammad to read, to which Muhammad replied, "I cannot," as he was not an educated man in that he had no prior schooling.

The angel then said to Muhammad: *"Read! in the Name of your Lord who created, created man from a clot of blood. Read! Your Lord is the most Bounteous, Who has taught the use of a pen, has taught mankind what he did not know"* (Qur'an 96:1–5).

This passage is important because it encourages the Muslim to read. But when we say 'read', we mean more than in the literal sense. It also means to think critically, to provoke thought. When you look at the Qur'anic scripture, you will notice that it always finishes by saying something along the lines of, "And this is for someone who thinks," "This is for the person who ponders," or "This is for the man of thought." It guides us not to believe in religion blindly, but to acknowledge the logic and science behind the teachings where science and logic exist, and where they do not, to seek or make the connection yourself.

Muhammad began preaching the revelations of Islam, claiming to be the prophet of God. According to Islamic tradition, Muhammad was the last of the prophets, following Jesus (Isa). The prophets were monotheists; they believed there was only one God. Prior to the advent of Islam, Arabs followed polytheism, worshipping multiple deities and idols in pagan Arabia.

Approximately one year after receiving the first revelation, Muhammad received the second. While waiting, he had developed a lack of certainty around what he had experienced. So much time had passed, and he still had not received the second revelation, but his wife, Khadijah, always supported and believed in him. When Muhammad finally received the second revelation, his doubts were put to rest.

One of the verses revealed to Muhammad forbade female infanticide and admonished those who would seek to carry out the despicable act. Essentially, one of the evilest acts associated with paganism at the time was now prohibited in the eyes of God.

The Prophet (PBUH) continued to spread his message for the next 13 years, attracting the slaves and the poor, and not so much the rich and famous. In Quraysh, an area in Mecca, his small number of followers became victims of abuse and torture. So, the Prophet, with his people, decided to flee to Medina to escape the oppression. When we reflect upon this, we see that the Prophet does not encourage us to stay and defend oppression. Instead, he implies that we have a right to physically remove ourselves from oppressive situations, whether they have been created by the government, our families, or the place where we live. Upon his arrival in Medina, the Prophet saw that the ecological conditions were far more conducive to a healthy life than what had been offered in Mecca.

As God continued delivering revelations to Muhammad (PBUH), the Qur'an began to include general guidelines and rules around nutrition, as well as marital relations, child rearing, and cleanliness. Any revelations that related to health, treatment, and hygiene, as well as Muhammad's own opinions on those matters, were collated and developed into a separate collection, titled *Tibb an-Nabī* (*Medicine of the Prophet*).

The Qur'an established the first relationship between nutrition and behaviour and the concepts of halal (meaning that with which is permissible) and tayyib (generally meaning wholesome, pure, organic, and clean). Many people think that the word 'halal' is a term limited to food, but this is incorrect. Anything can be labelled halal so long as it is permissible under Islamic law. We talk more about this in chapter six.

The Prophet provided the foundation of medicine and medical tradition that considers the human being in its totality, connecting the mind, body, and soul to the external environment by outlining specific instructions on various aspects of healthcare. He championed the interconnectivity between the physical, psychological, and spiritual spheres, claiming that health is more than simply maintaining the physical vessel.

When we consider medicine as it is today, we can see how much has changed over the last 1,400 years. Our modern healthcare practices follow a linear paradigm that focuses on the body alone and disconnects the spirit and environment from the human. We talk more about this in chapter two.

Prophetic Medicine is Based on Logic

Most prophetic medicine is based on logic because, generally, good health has always been the result of what is *logical* and *ethical*.

For example, when considering foods, the ancient Arabs could only consume crops that were able to grow locally under desert conditions. If merchants from Syria or Egypt brought food – they visited in caravans once or twice per year – Arabs could eat this too. Otherwise, diet was completely made up of foods that grew locally and were conducive to the soil and weather conditions of the area. Therefore, they ate almost entirely what grew in season, which resonates with the needs of the human body.

When we consider ancient history, we understand what sort of food should be consumed from an Islamic perspective. We acknowledge that whatever is in season – the way God designed and delegated it to be – is what we should be eating. Think about it. Garlic grows in autumn and winter because it helps our immune system and assists the body's detoxification processes. Then, spring and summer bring foods that are more antioxidant-rich and cooling to the body. There are divine reasons why these foods are available to us at certain times. The basic principle of eating in season is intuitive enough to help us recognise what to eat and when. If you asked, "What do I eat in summer?" The simple answer would be, "Whatever grows in summer in your local land."

Eating primarily foods that are in season can be challenging now that we have hybrids and the ability to import any fruit or vegetable from any part of the world. Although this provides an amazing opportunity for the modern man to eat and drink what he wants, it also creates a plethora of issues, including pollution during transportation, use of synthetic chemicals to preserve the food, issues with sustainability and effects on climate, and unjust food prices that create a larger gap between classes in terms of their ability to access foods. When considering the big picture, I do not believe the pros outweigh the cons.

Of course, in modern times, understanding the best produce to consume at any given time can be challenging. In Australia, it is sometimes difficult to determine what is in season. We have access to strawberries in winter and garlic in summer. Produce is perpetually available whereas in the time of the Prophet (PBUH), Arabs only had access to whatever grew under drought- or desert-like conditions. Although having a wider variety of food types available year-round may seem like a blessing, we must consider the ramifications for human health and the environment.

Vegetation was another important aspect of prophetic medicine. In the Arabian region, plants are primarily xerophyte, meaning they grow under dry conditions. Their roots spread deep underground, and they are capable of withstanding long periods of drought.

Across the Arabian Peninsula, date palms grew in the desert, along with other fruits and vegetables, including wheat, rice, alfalfa, barley, citrus, melons, tomatoes, and onions. In the higher regions, other fruit, including peaches and grapes, was available.[8] The ancient Arabs learned to leverage what was locally available to them, which usually meant food that was in season and able to thrive in dry desert conditions.

Due to the growth of certain vegetation in the region, Arabia was known for its production of frankincense.[9] Hadith, a collection of sayings from the Prophet (PBUH), acknowledge the use of the aromatic resin for a variety of health conditions, including those that involve inflammation, such as irritable bowel syndrome, as frankincense has antimicrobial properties for bacteria-related illnesses and reduction of rheumatism symptoms.[10]

Modern scientific literature corroborates these claims, with studies finding that frankincense has immune-modulating properties.[11] Not only can it stimulate a suppressed immune system, but it can help modulate an overactive immune response related to allergies, food intolerances, and other triggers. When the immune system overreacts, conditions such as eczema and psoriasis can occur. Because frankincense is capable of curbing this overreaction, it can be a powerful remedy for those suffering from certain disorders.

Frankincense is just one tool the Prophet identified all those centuries ago. Evidently, prophetic medicine understood back then what modern science is only rediscovering now. While we may have a deeper understanding of the mechanisms behind certain remedies, the results are still the same.

A Story of Sickness and Health

I will tell a story that puts into perspective the importance of the environment and overall health in preventing disease.

One of the kings in Persia sent Muhammad (PBUH) a learned physician. The physician remained in Arabia for one or two years, but no one ever approached him or sought his treatment. At last, he presented himself before the Prophet and complained, "I've been sent to treat you and your companions but during all this time, no one has asked me to carry out my duties in any respect whatsoever."

The Prophet replied, "It is the custom of these people to not eat until hunger overcomes them and to seize eating while there still remains a desire for food."

The physician answered, "This is the reason for their perfect health." Then he kissed the ground in reverence and departed.

This story highlights how the environment, our connection to the soil, the sun and the moon, eating in season, and having good mental health have an undeniable connection to good health overall. When we compare this to our current lifestyles, we see that we lack adequate sun exposure due to being stuck indoors, working 9–5 jobs. We hardly ever walk outside with our shoes off, let alone have gardens that allow us to do this. We spend a large amount of the night – if not all of it – indoors, absent of moonlight. Then we wonder why our mental and physical health deteriorates. We are disconnected from our environment, but we and it are in fact one, and we cannot exist without it.

Prophet Muhammad (PBUH) discusses food consumption in a Hadith: "The son of Adam does not fill any vessel worse than his stomach. It is enough for the son of Adam to eat a few mouthfuls to straighten his back, but if he must fill his stomach, then one third for his food, one third for his drink, and one third for his breath."[12]

The lesson from this is that, firstly, the upper limit of food consumption conducive to good health is literally only one third of your stomach, and the lower limit – the minimum we should eat – is enough to keep your back straight. It is a morsel of food, meaning just enough to grant you the energy to do your daily duties.

The issue is that our lifestyles and food consumption habits stray far from this suggestion. We consume excessively, and we eat for reasons other than hunger. Often, we eat for pleasure and comfort as well – for emotional reasons. Our diets are predominantly packaged foods, which are full of chemicals, preservatives, and pesticides, and much of it is likely eaten out of season.

We don't eat as many fruits and vegetables as we should. Our food has become hybrid, and our soils are depleted of important minerals and laced with carcinogenic herbicides and pesticides. Modern man is exposed to so many chemicals, and his poor liver and other detox organs are working overtime – and often they struggle. All of this comes together in a perfect storm that keeps man unwell and in a state of disease. It is challenging to say that a physically unwell human can have a deep-rooted connection with God. For that connection to be holistic, good physical health is a requirement.

Psychological Foundations of Islam

Islamic psychology stems from the concepts of the *nafs*, which is essentially the self – or the ego. Working on the ego and the heart in unison is an integral part of Islamic psychology. The heart is not just something that pumps blood throughout the body; it represents the entire human in relation to the world, as well as the approaching reality that we call the afterlife. A union exists between body and spirit. However, even in Islam, there is a lot about the spirit we do not know. To truly achieve good health, we must maintain the mind, body, and soul connection. We cannot disconnect our psychological health from the other aspects of our being, as all aspects of ourselves are deeply interconnected.

When we allow the vital forces of the body to become unbalanced, we create space for the manifestation of illness. The mental and psychological components of self can have a profound effect on the physical. For example, conventional medicine treats hypothyroidism with medications, such as levothyroxine, to address a deficiency in the hormone required for adequate thyroid function. As a result of this dysfunction, other symptoms and health complications emerge, which is why medical intervention and treatment is often necessary.

However, with a holistic approach, we do not simply acknowledge the deficiency and treat it with medication – we also seek the root cause. In my clinic, I regularly assist people with poor gut function that causes the small intestine to inadequately absorb nutrients. Iodine is essential for creating the thyroid hormone, and low absorption can produce a deficiency that translates to impaired thyroid function. By treating the cause – in this example, poor absorption of nutrients in the small intestine – and not just the symptoms, we can work towards fixing the problem rather than masking it with medication.

When examining this condition from a psychological perspective, we view the root cause as something else entirely. For example, low thyroid function could be the result of a person's inability to self-express. Because the thyroid is in the neck, dysfunction can represent a blockage in the energy channel that flows to the mouth. Therefore, to heal thyroid illness – other than by treating the iodine deficiency – we must allow the patient to find their voice and reclaim the ability to genuinely and authentically self-express. They must first recover from their psychological oppression before they can truly resolve any physical manifestations.

When we examine childhood trauma in relation to hypothyroidism, verbal or physical oppression is rarely the cause. We can also feel oppressed when we seek to fulfill a need to be loved. When we fail to receive unconditional love, we mould ourselves into models of who we think we need to be in order to receive – or even deserve – that which we lack.

The effects of such oppression on the organs are difficult to quantify scientifically. However, we must consider the emotional and spiritual realities as well as the physical. When we cannot be our authentic selves, it affects the throat chakra, and we may not even be aware because we have worn a mask our entire lives. It is what we thought we needed to do. It is where we thought we needed to be. But, eventually, the effects of lifelong oppression catch up with us, and we must either address the underlying issue or continue to suffer both mentally and physically.

In such cases, recovery requires significant psychological healing. However, many people view this approach as pseudoscientific, mostly because the science has not yet caught up. Because man's mind is so restricted and moulded in a certain way, thinking outside of the usual paradigm is challenging.

Constipation is another example of emotional issues manifesting physical conditions. When we are constipated, the physical cause may be a lack of beneficial bacteria, a fibre deficiency, poor movement of the muscles and contraction of the colon, elevated stress levels causing cortisol to reduce colonic movement, or a diet high in refined carbs and deficient in other elements. However, psychological and spiritual factors can also contribute to the problem. While we never deny the physical elements – they most certainly exist – we aim to treat each complaint holistically, considering all facets of the problem. In the case of constipation, the inability to emotionally 'let go' manifests as being physically unable to do the same. To adequately address the physical condition, we must also treat the underlying psychological cause.

As another example, cardiovascular disease is not just the result of a diet full of meat and dairy, cholesterol clogging the arteries, or a high-stress lifestyle lacking in movement. While these factors can contribute to cardiovascular disease on a physical level, a spiritual component also exists. Our hearts are unwell because they are in a void of spiritual presence, and they are neglected. The spiritual self cannot be healed through material means, and we cannot treat the infinite using finite resources. Only spirituality can offer infinite healing.

Cardiovascular disease is the leading cause of death in humans – and why is this?[13] Because the heart suffers so much sorrow in its inauthentic form. We die because of sadness. Disease cultivates within us, but we only seek to understand it in ways we can measure. However, not everything in life is quantifiable, and disease occurs when the spiritual self is misaligned with its purpose of creation.

Science now acknowledges that physical problems that manifest in the body can have emotional roots. In my clinic, I frequently see women who are undergoing premature menopause or experiencing ovarian failure, shorter cycles, or polycystic ovarian disease. Often, these women have suffered sexual trauma, either through rape or being in an unwanted relationship, unwillingly giving their bodies to their partners or husbands. Diseases of the reproductive tract can manifest from emotional problems linked to one of the most sacred things we do. If we knew the extent to which we transferred energy through sexuality, we would be extremely cautious about whom we opened our sexual energy channels to.

Establishing such an intimate connection with someone not only affects us emotionally, but also physically. I am not speaking of sexually transmitted infections; I mean the physical change in the uterine microbiome when exposed to someone else's microbiome and the long-term implications for our health and DNA.

For too long, we have denied the importance of the mind, body, and soul connection and its influence on health. We often consider it within a linear paradigm that disregards a significant portion of reality: our spiritual wellness.

CHAPTER TWO

TREATING THE BODY HOLISTICALLY

Have you heard the parable about the blind men and the elephant?

A group of five blind men heard that an elephant, an animal they were unfamiliar with, had been brought into town. Curious to learn more about the strange creature, the men decided to examine it by touch. Once they had located the elephant, they each reached out and began their examination.

The first man's hand landed on the trunk. "The elephant is very much like a snake," he said.

The second man's hand touched an ear. "No, the elephant more resembles a fan."

The third man's hand brushed a leg. "You're both wrong. The elephant is like a thick tree trunk."

The fourth man laid a hand on the elephant's side. "The elephant is clearly big and sturdy like a wall."

Finally, the fifth man touched a tusk. "Nonsense, the elephant is smooth and slender like a spear."

In life, we often fall victim to cases like this, as our exposure and understanding – or lack thereof – influences our comprehension. As humans, we tend to trust our own narrow perspectives, failing to see the bigger picture, the whole picture, the holistic picture, and instead having a very linear focus.

Linear medicine bears the same problem. Like in the parable about the elephant, we often lose perspective on what is actually going on when we solely focus on the symptom that the body is showing. The symptom, in essence, is the red flag the body has raised. The symptom is not the problem; it is just the alarm. The problem is deep and complex, and the symptom is just one branch of it, like the ear is just one part of the elephant. When we view each organ as a mechanical piece of flesh and disassociate the organs from one another, when we are blinded to the orchestra of work the organs do through communicating with one another, we are merely as blind as the men in the parable, who view the elephant incompletely.

Think about it. Skin irritation? See a dermatologist, who deals with the skin only. Hormones out of whack? Perhaps a gynaecologist or an endocrinologist may offer a solution. There is a specialist for everything. I am not suggesting that medical experts are dispensable – their work is paramount – just that their focus is to only treat the issues relevant to their area of practice, dismissing any connection to any other organ. In fact, the reality is that more often than not, the symptom presenting in one organ is due to another's lack of function. The idea should be to treat the human, not the symptom nor the condition's label – but many of us do not operate this way. We treat the symptom because, in linear medicine, the goal is to keep someone alive, not necessarily to improve their quality of life.

Instead, if we have polycystic ovaries, we see a gynaecologist. If we have thyroid problems, which commonly accompanies polycystic ovaries, we see an endocrinologist. If we have mental health issues due to the resulting hormone imbalance, we see a psychologist or psychiatrist and potentially get medicated. However, all of these organs work in synergy with one another. The hypothalamus, the thyroid, the adrenals, and the ovaries all work together to regulate sex and stress hormone production. When we see a different specialist for each symptom, we replicate the blind men's approach to the elephant.

The small intestine is the governing factory of neurotransmitters, the hormones that control our mood. But when our mood is down, we don't look to treat the gastrointestinal system. No one asks us to seek help for our small intestine or explore the connection between poor gut function and poor mental health. Instead, we treat the symptom of the mental health challenge as 'depression', masking it with antidepressants. Again, not to say there is no place for this. However, we have got to a place where our focus on treating symptoms has led to a plethora of people feeling hopeless and powerless, blaming genetics and, thus, relying only on external sources for healing. Like Rumi says: "The wound is the place where the Light enters you." However, for decades, we have been masking pain. We have been masking discomfort because we have not been taught how to engage with it, what its real job is, and why it is there. We prefer to disconnect from anything that feels uncomfortable, foreign, or displaced.

The Western ideology of medicine does not so much focus on causes; it mainly seems to care about the currently affected organ and band-aid solutions that allow the human body to continue to function with a crutch for the rest of its life. With illnesses skyrocketing, it is fair to want to keep people alive at all costs, often sacrificing quality of life for continued life. But when will we as practitioners place the responsibility of health back onto the shoulders of the individual? When will we stop relying on drugs and temporary solutions that mask rather than cure? When will we consider the entire elephant? When will we allow for the creation of a responsible, conscious society as the Qur'an mentions? When will we allow the vicegerents of the Earth to take back their power and control?

You may not be responsible for the outcome, but you are certainly responsible for the journey.

Seeing the Elephant

When we view symptoms in isolation, treatment cannot be as effective as it would if we considered the situation through a holistic lens. Modern medicine needs to recalibrate the way it administers treatment and focus on healing the *cause* of the illness, infection, or imbalance rather than simply addressing the symptoms.

Up until around 100 years ago, many masters and medical doctors focused on treating the cause of a complaint; aligning the human body's physical and spiritual needs; connecting man to nature, the sun, and the moon; treating the person as a whole, and acting as a teacher, educating the individual on how to heal and, once healed, how to stay well. A century ago, this was the standard treatment and when I look at how far we have come, I wonder whether we have progressed or *re*gressed. In some areas, regression is certainly evident.

Yes, we create solutions. But are we also creating additional problems? For example, there are now some great cancer therapy options; however, in our pursuit to find an effective treatment, did we ever stop and think about removing carcinogenic chemicals from our foods, our cleaning products, and our environment? Did we tell women about the possible link between conventional underarm deodorant laced with aluminium and an increased risk of developing breast cancer (while we allowed these very same companies to use the pink ribbon, unbeknown to us that it is also the chemicals in their products that may cause the very problem they are proclaiming to care about)?[14] Did we tell them that the make-up that leaves their skin so flawless can contain heavy metals that are known to be carcinogenic?[15] Have we invested even 5 percent of the money we pile into cancer research in cancer prevention? If we took a preventative approach, how different would future cancer rates be?

When we have a headache, we rarely stop and consider the cause. Why? Because we can simply take a pill to make the pain go away. But discomfort is a sign, a signal from the body that something is wrong. In our high-paced lives, we do not want to consider the whys. The whys take too much time, money, and effort. It is much easier to ask, "What will relieve me from this pain or discomfort right now?" Often, the answer is a pill, a medicine, a quick but temporary fix, which certainly comes with long-term consequences. You don't just take a painkiller for pain relief and assume that it comes into your body, takes away your pain with rainbows and butterflies, and leaves your body with no further ado. It takes a lot of effort by the liver to break down the medication and then to excrete it. Sometimes, it succeeds; other times, it does not. And when it does not, we experience side effects.

Many medications have undesirable side effects. For instance, we do not often worry about how the non-steroidal anti-inflammatories we take affect gut integrity and function. We do not have time for that. We would prefer to block the message because we do not have time to acknowledge what our bodies are trying to tell us. What *do* we have time for, then?

Your headache may be the result of dehydration, stress, muscle tension, excessive caffeine use, magnesium deficiency, lack of oxygen due to allergies, high levels of mercury or aluminium, a dormant viral infection, a brain tumour – the list of possible causes is endless. However, you will never learn the cause by masking the symptoms and if you do not address the source of the problem, the affliction – in this case, the headache – will likely return. If you continue to medicate, the cycle repeats until the treatment triggers another symptom, another ailment, another bodily signal you may be able to mask with more medication. Inevitably, more side effects emerge, which require more medication to manage, and the cycle goes on and on until the body can no longer cope. Eventually, what seemed like a simple headache in the beginning can transform into a chronic illness that you can no longer ignore or simply put a band-aid on, and perhaps you continue to do exactly that – at the cost of your quality of life.

I am not suggesting that taking pain relief for a headache is wrong; sometimes it is the only way you can continue with your day, especially when you have a plethora of responsibilities you cannot ignore. However, we must consider the body *as a whole* if we want to experience our best physical and mental selves. Short-term solutions may keep us going, keep us alive, but they will not allow us to live our lives to our full potential. If we bury our heads in the sand regarding our own chronic health challenges, how can we connect to the Creator through conscious living, especially when we can barely get through the day?

How many times have you sighed because you needed to perform your ablution again because you kept breaking wind thanks to that doughnut you had for lunch? Or you've missed morning prayer again because your body was working excessively hard while you slept to break down the build-up of toxins from the chronic inflammation contributed by your diet? Or how you struggle to fast and cannot see past the struggle of caffeine withdrawal, and, between you and me, your deepest darkest secret is that while everyone celebrates the coming of the month of fasting, you cannot wait for it to be over because the struggle is real?

The same applies when we are trying to lose weight. We nearly kill ourselves attempting to stick to fad diets and strenuous exercise regimes to shift the kilos. We are so focused on wanting to lose weight because that is the only way we know how to love ourselves. Often, we feel that unless we are thinner, the self-hate cycle will continue. In the short-term, this approach might work but if the mindset that created the anomaly in the physical body is not resolved, we will struggle to keep the weight off long-term. We must work on the mindset that created the connection with food that compels us to use it as medical analgesia. It numbs us. It helps us live another day on this earth plane without needing to dig deep into our wounds, without allowing our shadows to creep up, without dealing with the mental health issues that created this poor relationship with food in the first place. Perhaps we feel as though eating is the only thing in life we have control over or we actually enjoy it short-term (because sugar and casein act as drugs that stimulate and numb the brain).

Unless we choose to dig deep, to face our shadows, to address our mental health, we could spend thousands of dollars on fads and shed thousands of tears looking for answers and mercy on the pages of social media, in the words of the next big influencer, when the answers and healing lie within. It is only when we break that we can receive light. If we keep bandaging the crack, that light will never get a chance to enter.

Bacteria, Viruses, and Fungi

*"It may be that you hate something when it is good for you
and it may be that you love something when it is bad for you.
Allah knows and you do not know."*
– Qur'an 2:216

For a long time, we have been pseudoscientific in our approach to bacteria, viruses, and fungi. Ever since man first stepped foot on Earth, these living organisms have been a normal part of our genome. They are a fundamental part of any healthy person. They make up our ecology and are important in preventing disease, more so than causing it, and only become a problem if there is an overgrowth, an imbalance, if our terrain is disturbed. Bacterial infections that we get labelled with, such as pneumonia, H. pylori, streptococcus, and staphylococcus, are all commensal, meaning they live in the body; they belong in the body; they serve a purpose. However, it is their overgrowth that contributes to problems. Therefore, we must ask: How do we keep the terrain clean to prevent illness? How do we live and eat to prevent overgrowth of these otherwise commensal organisms? What are the things in our environments that are affecting the balance, the otherwise finely orchestrated community of microbes that belong?

In 1931, Otto Warburg was awarded the Nobel Prize in Physiology or Medicine for his work on the aerobic and anaerobic metabolic process in cells. His work had massive implications for our understanding of cancer. Dr Warburg asserts that, "The prime cause of cancer is the replacement of the respiration of oxygen in normal body cells by a fermentation of sugar."[16] Fermentation is an anaerobic process, meaning it does not require oxygen, and Dr Warburg discovered that cancer cells can survive and develop without it. Later studies revealed that flooding the body with oxygen using hyperbaric treatment may inhibit the development of some cancer subtypes.[17] Slightly alkaline blood is the ideal pH for oxygenation, and our blood naturally exists in an alkaline state.[18] So, does this mean that maintaining alkalinity and high oxygen levels can inhibit certain cancers?

Dr Warburg's research led others to theorise that anaerobic bacteria, yeast, fungi, and cancer cells cannot survive, multiply, or take over cells in a highly oxygenated environment.[19] This belief is known as 'terrain theory' and focuses on the part the body plays in handling infection and disease. For too long, we have worshipped the germ theory, but that is only one piece of the overarching health puzzle. Why not try looking at the world with a new set of glasses? Perhaps you will see things a little clearer. Both germ and terrain theories are scientifically valid and worthy of our attention. However, I would underline that they are still both only theories.

For too long, we have viewed bacteria as boogie monsters when, in fact, we each have approximately 200 g of bacteria in our bodies, working in synergy to help us absorb nutrients, make amino acids, help the organs communicate with one another, and perform other vital tasks.[20] Without these crucial bacterial colonies, the human body would not function. This is why we use faecal microbial transplants (FMT) to treat gastrointestinal autoimmune illnesses, such as ulcerative colitis and Crohn's. Research suggests that deficiencies in – not an excess of – different colonies of bacteria may contribute to these chronic illnesses.[21] Additionally, *Lactobacillus rhamnosus* is often used to treat children exhibiting symptoms of eczema, as a deficiency in this bacterial strain can cause or exacerbate the condition.[22]

Ample evidence exists to suggest that a deficiency of bacteria can contribute to other autoimmune disorders, which is why new science is being developed that looks at FMT to treat autoimmune diseases. The treatment involves removing a healthy person's stool and placing it into a patient's body. The bacteria in the stool reinoculate the microbiome and switch off certain genes that code for autoimmune illnesses or prevent the switching on of those that code for autoimmunity.[23]

So, why are we so quick to declare bacteria our enemy? Why do we so easily turn a blind eye to all other possible causes and contributing factors to ill health? Why are we still ignoring the growing body of evidence that allows us to better understand why when two different people experience the same disease type, one can heal quite quickly, and the other may experience a longer healing time and more complications when the offending agent is the same?

Wonders and Risks of Antibiotics

When penicillin was discovered in 1928, the world was entranced. The 'wonder drug' was revolutionary, saving the lives of countless people, and was used widely in the treatment of soldiers during World War II. Since then, antibiotics have continued to be developed – albeit to a lesser extent in the last 30 years – and have almost eliminated many previously life-threatening infections. Thanks to antibiotics, we generally no longer need to worry about infections like syphilis, bronchitis, or pneumonia killing us.

Although the discovery and development of antibiotics has been groundbreaking, society's obsession with the treatment has caused us to form exaggerated beliefs about its superpower properties. We incorrectly assume it can cure any ailment that comes our way. We take antibiotics for almost everything. When we have an infection – regardless of whether it is viral-, fungal-, or exosome-related – we are usually prescribed a round of antibiotics to reduce the bacterial load in the system. Antibiotics offer peace of mind, both for the doctor administering them and the patient ingesting them. From their perspectives, the harm caused by the infection outweighs the side effects of taking antibiotics unnecessarily.

Recently, I was at the pharmacy, getting some documents verified, when I overheard the conversation the lady in front of me was having with the lady at reception. "I've taken three days of my antibiotics, however, I still have the issue, so can I just get another prescription for another three days?" The lady at reception said there was no need and that three days was ample. However, the customer insisted. The pharmacist ended up suggesting the use of an antifungal in the interim and for her to see her doctor if the symptoms persisted. So, she was pretty much taking antibiotics for what she assumed was bacterial, and then was given an antifungal. I am so confused right now. The overuse of antibiotics is costing us as much as what it was costing us to not have antibiotics in the first place. Let me elaborate further.

Accumulating evidence challenges the haphazard approach of overprescribing antibiotics. For the most part, we are not dying of bacteria-related illnesses as much anymore, but a disproportionate number of people do have their quality of life decreased significantly due to autoimmune diseases, where the immune cells of the body attack its own tissue as it loses its ability to recognise friend from foe. Research suggests that excessive use of antibiotics is one of the drivers for such reactions in children.[24]

Improper use of antibiotics can cause a long-term detriment to the human body and ecology of the world. In the body, antibiotics can create microbial imbalances and ruin the cohesion of the microbiome with the human genome.[25] Due to their inability to distinguish between what they need to kill versus what needs to stay – what we incorrectly refer to as 'good' and 'bad' bacteria – antibiotics can kill off healthy colonies that would otherwise keep infection at bay, facilitate the absorption of nutrients, and act as messengers between organs. Often, we are confused about whether the issue is with the wild strain, the mutated strains due to overexposure of antibiotics, or the disruption in the terrain, which allows for the overgrowth in the first place.

We have collectively misused and overused antibiotics to the point where bacteria are becoming increasingly antibiotic resistant. Instead of being killed by antibiotics, more and more bacteria modify their genetics to survive treatment. Furthermore, superbugs, such as *E. coli* (H30-Rx strain), have become so intelligent that they have developed many different defence mechanisms to prevent dying post exposure to antibiotics.[26] This makes treatment of these infections exceedingly difficult and expensive and potentially brings us back to square one: a pre-antibiotic era where people were dying of otherwise preventable diseases. Now, due to antibiotic resistance, certain bacteria are not only not responding to antibiotics, but they are also changing their DNA to create tougher genetic material, making them harder to treat via natural methods too.[27] So, does this mean we are almost at square one again?

I do not deny the lifesaving effects of antibiotics in appropriate situations. The challenge is that pseudoscience still sees bacteria as the bad guy, leading to overexposure and overuse of the drug – for example, a doctor prescribing antibiotics without thoroughly checking a patient's symptoms. As a result, we create more opportunity for autoimmunity and thrush, a very common side effect of antibiotic exposure, as defeated bacterial strains allow the liberation of candida, which takes off exponentially.[28]

Again, I am not suggesting that antibiotics should not be used – on the contrary. In order that they continue to save lives, we should be more diligent with how often we prescribe them so we are not left with excessively powerful superbugs that are detrimental to the quality and quantity of the lives of our loved ones.

A client of mine had an ill child – runny nose, fever, vomiting, ear infections, swollen adenoids and tonsils, the works – who had been prescribed antibiotics to treat the condition, on not just one but many occasions. Despite the drugs, the child continued to get sick, to the point where he became chronically ill every month. The mother had no idea what to do. Her child had been prescribed every antibiotic under the sun, and yet nothing was working.

As soon as the mother came to me, I knew that one of two things had occurred: either the child had developed a resistance to the antibiotics, or they had been prescribed incorrectly. After all, the child's sickness could have originated from a virus, parasite, protozoa, or cellular cleansing. It could have come from anything *but* bacteria. However, because the linear model of medicine typically administers the antibiotic first, that was the treatment he received. "If it works, then it's bacteria. If it doesn't, it's a virus, so go and rest."

This is far from being an argument about whether natural medicine is better than conventional. Look at the bigger picture. This is about ensuring that severely mutated bacterial strains don't occur. It is about reducing the load on our healthcare system and our healthcare workers. It is about improving our quality of life so we don't spend our lives with our heads stuck in the sand and we have a chance to pursue helping others and being conscious in our consumption and use of the earth plane.

Now, just because someone has contracted a virus, it does not mean that there are no treatment options. Supplements that contain herbs, vitamins, minerals, and extracts, such as echinacea, astragalus, vitamin C, zinc, and elderberry, can fight off infection by increasing the body's white blood cell count.[29] This is our innate immunity. The increase in white blood cells helps to ward off whatever is making the patient sick by stimulating the immune system, which was put there by the Creator. The one who created man also created his immune system, with no fault upon creation. However, chronic exposure to untested chemicals from our foods, soils, and environment, chronic nutritional deficiencies, electromagnetic fields (EMFs), heavy metal exposure, plastics, and many other factors have led us to suffer from severe immune compromise, making our immune systems less effective than they should be. For example, there have been deletions in gene pathways that cleanse the liver through glutathione.[30] How did that gene deletion occur? How did we lose much of our ability to detoxify over the years? Could these untested and undertested chemicals have anything to do with it? Evidence suggests this might be the case.[31] I think; therefore I am. Or I am; therefore I think?

I suggested that my client give her child a powdered supplement that encouraged the production of white blood cells due to the herbs and vitamins included. Additionally, herbs and nutraceuticals in the remedy would kill off bacterial overgrowth, deal with viruses and exosome cleansing, and assist with rehydration. When you are sick, your immune system does not want to deal with digesting food. Digesting costs too much energy, and, at that stage, the body needs to invest all the energy it can into healing. Therefore, it prefers to conserve energy for this.

As a matter of fact, in Islamic medicine, Tirmidhi reported that Uqbah ibn Amir al-Juhani said that "The Messenger of Allah (blessings and peace of Allah be upon him) said: 'Do not force your sick ones to eat or drink. Allah will feed them and give them to drink'." In our very own backyard, it tells us not to force-feed our sick. 1400 years ago, we were given this information, and here we are still forcing chicken noodle soup and other foods down the throat of people who are unwell.

Now, let us go back to my patient, the child. As the child was experiencing a fever, we also needed to safeguard against him reaching a temperature that would trigger a febrile convulsion. Not that convulsions are dangerous per se, but they freak us out, and we would much prefer that the body regulate the highs and lows of the fever. The fever was not the enemy; it just meant that the immune system was working by heating up the body to kill off the problematic pathogen or chemical. It is the fever that denatures the viral proteins. The fever 'burns' off the toxins, so we are happy to still preserve and safeguard the speed of the rise in temperature. The mother was to check in on the child every 30 minutes and if there was a spike, every five minutes to ensure that the rise was only temporary and the body was modulating and navigating through it fine. Fever-reducing medication was available if the intervention was warranted. The issue, though, with fever-reducing medication is that it interferes with a very natural process, given and designed by the divine to help the body ward off whatever is manipulating its homeostasis.

Within 24 to 32 hours, the fever was completely gone, which could be translated to: the body had rid itself of the very thing it needed to denature or disarm. The body was creating mucus – a sign that the bacteria, virus, or exosome was being expelled – and the child's appetite returned. By stimulating the child's immune system, rather than pumping it with antibiotics, the body was strong enough to work through the illness and stave off the infection. So, rather than relying on an external helper, such as antibiotics, we instead turned inward and switched on the immune function to heal the body. In natural medicine, using supplements or herbs that are anti-microbial helps treat the infection primarily by killing infection-causing bacteria and secondarily by supporting the immune system to make more white blood cells for the immune and detox processes.

If we work *with* the body and listen to what it needs, we can achieve better short- and long-term health for ourselves and others. Not only will gentle treatment options assist the body in curing itself, reserving antibiotic use for relevant conditions will help them remain a lifesaving tool.

However, if we keep using antibiotics unnecessarily – for example, at the first sign of a cold or flu – bugs will continually evolve and become less responsive to treatment. This could mean losing lives to infections that would otherwise have been treated with antibiotics as they were less than a century ago.

God's Cure for All

The last prophet of Islam, Prophet Muhammad, may peace be upon Him, tells us there is a cure to all illnesses and diseases, except for death. I see that we struggle to see that the cure is in the immune system and the natural ecology of the Earth, in herbs, spices, and vitamins, somewhere in nature (mostly where they have told us not to look). In my opinion, it is not necessarily in a man-made drug. However, few businesses want to invest money in something that cannot be patented. For example, you cannot patent the poppy; however, heroin, morphine, and other such opiates trace their origins to this single plant. It has been cultivated for centuries, and the only way to patent it and make money is to copy its chemical structure and develop a synthetic version. It is going to sound so cheesy, but there is no money in health; there is no money in cures; there is no profit in creating a society full of robust, healthy, wise humans with great longevity.

Look around and tell me if you see anything that has originated from anything without first originating from God, aka nature? What do I mean by this? Let us use colours as an example. Has man ever come up with a colour that was not already on the Earth, bearing witness through a flower, an insect, or a plant? Has man ever come up with anything that was not initially taken from the creation of God?

The doctrine of signatures is an old natural philosophy suggesting that the outward appearance of a thing's body indicates its special healing properties and that there is a relationship between the outward qualities of medicinal objects and the disease, the inadequacies they are to heal. So, it is literally God's fingerprint. For instance, chestnuts are good for the brain, but they also *look* like the brain. Similarly, the outside of a walnut resembles the wrinkles and folds of the brain's neocortex. Carefully crack open a walnut, and you will see two sides, left and right. These represent the left and right hemispheres of the brain. Notice the thin part in between. This represents the brain's corpus callosum, which divides, or bridges, each side. Look closely at the nut, and you can even detect upper and lower cerebellums.

Walnuts contain high amounts of gallic and ellagic acid, two antioxidants that increase in concentration when cooked. They also contain antioxidants and minerals, like magnesium and potassium, that help reduce the risk of cardiovascular issues, such as heart disease or stroke. Additionally, walnuts contain high amounts of omega-3 fatty acids, which feed the brain. Because the brain is around 60 percent fat, omega-3 is one the most crucial molecules for determining its integrity and capacity to perform.[32]

Let us explore a few more examples. Carrots resemble the human eye and are very high in vitamin A, one of the most important vitamins for eye health. Tomatoes have four chambers and are red like our hearts. They also have a high amount of lycopene, which protects the heart against oxidative damage. Celery, bok choy, rhubarb – all these linear plants look like bones and contain so many minerals that are important for bone health. Onions look like cells when sliced and act like a Roto-Rooter system by clearing waste materials from our cells and bodies. This is why onions are important for winter – not only because they are antimicrobial but also because we get sicker at that time of year. We show symptoms in the beginning of winter and autumn because, like nature, our bodies too are cleansing and detoxing. Just like the trees that lose their leaves, our bodies during autumn and winter lose their degenerated cells. They clear out unwanted, dodgy, useless, and otherwise disease-causing cells through a natural cleansing process and by releasing what are called exosomes, which resemble viruses.[33]

When cells cleanse, they release exosomes, which are tiny vesicles that contain DNA, RNA, and other waste material.[34] Initially, we are detoxing and, thus, have symptoms of illness. When this process is interrupted or the body cannot adequately clear waste matter from the cells, toxins may get stuck, circulating in the blood because drainage pathways, such as the bowels, are blocked. The excessive liberation of these toxins into the circulatory system causes symptoms of illness that then translate to fungal or bacterial overgrowth when we allow the waste material to linger in the blood for too long. At this point, we usually reach for antibiotics or require drug intervention to heal.

These natural processes were the very first things that granted man some clues during his quest for wisdom and knowledge in the life sciences. As I mentioned earlier, Islamic medicine is mostly built on logic. However, man's ego got in the way, and he forgot that the brain he was using to understand life was given to him by the Creator;thus, his capacity to comprehend was limited to what God allowed.

Pain – to Feel or Not to Feel

Our approach to pain is similar to our approach to germs. When we feel discomfort, we run for the pain-relief drug. Why? Because we have not been taught to acknowledge and welcome pain and discomfort as messengers of the body who are grieving and trying to tell us what needs assistance. Instead, we prefer to shoot the messenger by silencing him with medication. Does this remove the problem? No. It simply band-aids the symptom. It may also create long-term issues, but we are not interested in the long-term; we are only interested in the now. So, when we shoot the messenger, we become more and more disconnected from our authentic selves and from the conscious ability to understand logically what the symptom is trying to tell us and, thus, what we actually need to do then and there.

As with antibiotics, there are times when we need to use pain medication. Even some of my patients use it while we address the drivers of their pain. Pain medication has a place, but it should not be the only avenue of treatment. We must always turn inwards and try to understand the *why* so we can treat the cause of the pain effectively.

In a nutshell, pain is a signal from an injured part of the body that travels through the nerves until it is registered by the brain. The body's immune system responds to the injury by creating its own treatment plan for the problem it has discovered – and sometimes it does not. Sometimes it cannot. Genetically, it knows it must restore homeostasis – this is embedded in its genetic potential by the best of creators – but due to swimming in a plethora of chemicals, toxins, and deficiencies in the microbiome, there is lack of communication between the brain and the injury. Therefore, as much as it tries to reach homeostasis, medical intervention is initially the only way out because the body is far too unwell to use its innate healing processes or for these processes to be 'good enough' at first to help the body out of distress.

It is going to sound like a far stretch but when we look at things holistically, we must also consider the emotional, lifestyle, and behavioural realities that brought us here. Many of us cannot tolerate pain because we are not able to sit in discomfort. I mean that many of us today cannot even sit on the toilet without our phones because of the subconscious fear of connecting to what may come up emotionally if our brains are not consistently engaged.

Part of our dislike for pain stems from our upbringing. Many of us, when we were children and fell and hurt our knees, scraped our elbows, or bumped our heads, did not have parents who hugged us and allowed us to feel our emotions through complaining or crying or screaming. A lot of our parents did not know how to deal with emotions themselves, so they rushed us through them by saying things like, "Sshh, it's not that bad. You're a big boy," or, "Big girls don't cry," or they redirected our behaviour before we had an opportunity to process the emotion. This translates to unhealed physical trauma manifesting in our bodies mentally and spiritually. No one really held space for us when we felt discomfort; they taught us to distract ourselves from it, belittle the experience, deny the pain, or ignore it. As a result, we grew up to be adults who cannot tolerate an ounce of physical pain, who do not know what to do other than dissociate and distract ourselves when we do have physical or mental symptoms that even slightly resemble anything painful or uncomfortable. We see pain as the bad guy, the enemy and not the messenger it actually is.

Let us pretend that you now have a bacterial infection because your terrain has been assaulted for so long. The infection creates pain and inflammation. The pain and inflammation trigger the immune system to migrate cells to the area of infection to treat it. This process also involves sending a message to the brain to alarm you to be conscious of what is happening so you can take further action. For example, you have pain in your ankle because it is sprained, so the physical messenger of pain is not just there to wake up internal healing mechanisms but also to act as an external protection mechanism to ensure that you are not stepping on that sprained leg. It is asking you to rest and slow down. God forbid, you take that advice!

Pain is a blessing in disguise. It gives us so much information prior to 'shutting off'. Pain tells us immediately that something is not right. It gives us clues to what could be wrong and what needs to be fixed. What an intelligent system! It notifies us of problems so we can respond. When we look at pain from a holistic, rather than linear, paradigm, pain suddenly serves the much greater purpose of awakening the body.

A client of mine was suffering from stage four endometriosis, a severe condition where the tissue inside the uterus grows outside of it, creating unbearable, chronic pain as one of many symptoms. The pain had completely encumbered her life, to the point where she could not work or complete basic tasks like cooking or cleaning. She could not even walk inside her home without wearing sneakers.

As part of her endometriosis treatment, she was injected with a hormone to stop her periods, leading her into perimenopause at the age of 36. She was put on hormone replacement therapy and would lock herself in her room for the ten days surrounding the period created by the synthetic estrogen and progesterone. For those ten days, she would not speak to anyone, including her two young children, because her pain and moods were so debilitating. This was her way of protecting her children from her unprecedented emotional wrath.

Of course, the endometriosis was the main driver of this woman's pain. However, what we needed to do was look at her problem holistically. We needed to listen to her body's signals to uncover whether anything else was contributing to her symptoms and, if so, how we could treat it. There was no point masking the pain with medication if we could resolve the secondary drivers. What else was her body alerting us to? What were some of the causes of endometriosis? How many slices did this pie have, and how could we uncover all the different causes and work on each one?

We started by investigating her gut health, which revealed that she was suffering from intestinal permeability. We then discovered undetected food intolerances and a bacterial infection in the small intestine. By simply identifying these three drivers, we were able to reduce her pain by about 30 percent. This enabled her to stop wearing shoes in the home.

As we continued exploring supplementary drivers of her chronic pain, I turned my attention to her cannabinoid pathway. Every person has a complex system within them – the endocannabinoid system – that helps manage various internal processes and acts as a chemical pathway in the brain.[35] Within this system are endogenous cannabinoids: lipids that can, among other things, regulate pain perception.[36] It seemed to me that her system was not functioning as it should. I prescribed her certain phytonutrients to reregulate the cycle of inflammation, and, amazingly, her pain reduced considerably. She was able to go back to work, which was very empowering because she had been financially relying on her husband. She could also resume doing the things she enjoyed and no longer experienced debilitating pain when she got her period – a hot water bottle and a cup of tea is now all she needs to keep comfortable. I certainly did a lot more to address the many other causes of her condition not mentioned here, but these examples are included to show you that it is hardly ever one thing that causes and creates a disease. Often, it is many different things that need to be addressed.

We currently work with conditions like endometriosis by acknowledging that it is not in fact a hormonal issue. It is the immune system of the uterus, which is responsible for excreting waste matter via endometrial lining each month, not working effectively. So, how can we understand why it is not working properly and enhance its performance? These are the types of questions we must ask.

By taking the time to explore what the body is telling us via its messenger – pain – we can alleviate symptoms *and* target the root of the problem. This is a much more effective strategy when trying to combat pain long-term. Rather than silencing our bodies, we need to actively listen to what they are telling us. This is the only way we can begin to achieve optimum health.

Pain in Labour

"And We have enjoined on man (to be dutiful and good) to his parents. His mother bore him in weakness and hardship upon weakness and hardship, and his weaning is in two years. Give thanks to Me and to your parents, unto Me is the final destination."
– Qur'an 31:14

There is no denying that giving birth is one of the most painful experiences a person can endure. Perhaps to say "the most discomforting" is a better phrase to use, but all we are really doing is sugar-coating and relabelling pain, which doesn't take away the feeling and emotion associated with it. Allah acknowledges that we are in a state of weakness and pain during labour, but the pain has a divine purpose – as a communicator and a blessing – and there will be ease and relief with it, not just at the end of it.

When we are in a state of contraction (I prefer to call this 'waves', as even now 'contraction' causes me to cringe), the first blessing is that the waves come and go. We are given a break as the pain goes from 100/10 one minute to zero the next, kind of like what happens in a fever naturally. The temperature fluctuates to cause discomfort to the pathogenic microbes and denature them, as they cannot withstand temperature fluctuations.

When we block out the pain with any form of pain management, we inhibit the body's ability to respond, communicate, and properly do what it needs to do: open up the uterus further and produce oxytocin (the 'love hormone'). Oxytocin assists the birth by moving the baby through the birthing canal and helps strengthen the connection between mother and child. When you stifle pain with an epidural, your body's production of oxytocin is lowered.[37] This can contribute to a longer labour due to the body not understanding well whether it is in labour or not and, thus, halting or getting confused in the steps it needs to take to bring the baby Earthside. You may also be unable to produce as much breastmilk, as there is no innate ability for the body to recognise it is birthing. In many cases, we have forced it into this state through induction, using something very similar to the hormone oxytocin that is not in fact oxytocin. As women, we tend to get very offended when anyone speaks of inductions and epidurals. I suppose, subconsciously, we feel a sense of guilt and shame around why we couldn't do it like the other women when, in fact, it is not us who has failed; the system has failed us. The system has left us disempowered because it tells us to trust it and others rather than trusting our gut instincts, our bodies, and our own selves.

We need to view labour as a natural part of becoming a mother, rather than a 'risky procedure' that requires medication and intervention. If we trust our bodies to deal with pain, they will be able to perform optimally. They have been doing this with no aid for centuries. The body has an innate genetic intelligence; it is engraved in our genes how birthing occurs, and we must place trust back in our bodies, look at the system, and allow it to be more woman-centred rather than hospital-centred. The body already knows how to birth. It is not something we need to teach it. We just have to stop intervening in relation to the natural discomfort and pain that occurs as a messenger to the plethora of hormonal synchrony that needs the pain messengers to be triggered. If we do not, our bodies will not function as intended. Stifling pain, particularly when it comes to labour, is a choice that should only be made after careful consideration. I would encourage anyone considering using pain management during labour to speak with a holistic obstetrician/gynaecologist, a holistic doula, midwife, or health practitioner to acknowledge all possible routes pre administration of any medication, as intervention will almost always breed more intervention.

Even though I had three medication-free labours, they were far from similar. With my firstborn, my daughter, I had no idea how to manage my breath, how to welcome discomfort, or how to listen to the cues of my body. Therefore, I suffered for six hours in agonising pain, using my body as a TENS machine. I bit my arm to distract myself from the pain. I dug my fingernails into my thighs, again, to distract my body from the pain, as a TENS machine would. All of this because I had no idea about using my breath to control the outcome and the intensity of pain. As a result, I had my beautiful daughter in my arms six hours later, but the trauma caused me to not talk about labour for five or six months. I would tear up at the thought of it. I had a profound resentment for labour, and my brain erased much of the experience from my memory.

In contrast, with my second born, my son, labour was just over an hour. At 10.45 pm, my body had an excessive urgency to open my bowels and empty them. After 10–20 minutes of constantly using the bathroom, I started getting waves – three waves in ten minutes. My husband filled the tub up with water to allow me to stay at home as long as possible. I was breathing through my waves and reciting affirmations. For me, these were religious affirmations that had come to me, in my opinion, through divine decree. I kept saying, "Inne meal usri Yusra," which translates in English to, "Verily there is relief with pain." I did not say it on purpose. I had not planned it or written it anywhere. It just came to me during the right time.

The waves genuinely felt like minor period pain. Through a hypno-birthing course, I had learned to control my breath and understood how oxygenating the blood via correct breathing altered my perception of pain and discomfort. This allowed the labour to speed up or, I should say, allowed the labour to occur in only as much time as it needed, not any more and not any less.

I told my husband we had to leave. I had a wave in the garage and in the car. When I arrived at the hospital, they wheeled me into the birthing room because there was no way I could walk. I was in active labour. My husband placed warm water on my back while I had waves in the shower. I breathed my way through each one and listened to when my body was ready to breathe.

At 1.05 am, I delivered my son. It was the most liberating feeling to be able to hold space for myself, to respect my own needs, and trust my body before I trusted anything else. I caught him in my hand and tears of joy and gratitude to the Creator poured down my face as I acknowledged and bore witness to the innate power he had blessed me with to make this miracle happen.

My third labour experience was similar to my second. The waves just felt like minor period pain, and I allowed myself to wholeheartedly feel everything I had to feel in that moment. I did nothing to distract myself and completely submitted to the divine intellectual and genetic capacity and capability of my body, the very body that had done it twice before through the will of God, and I had the most amazing 2.5-hour labour. I will never forget the moment my daughter stared at me, completely alert. I had never felt so connected with God as I did in those very moments of discomfort and pain.

Treating the Cause

If you opened the Qur'an at page one and read it through to the end, it would not read like a book with a beginning, middle, and end. The Qur'an is holistic by nature. We cannot extract a verse and translate it in isolation, just like we cannot take a passage from the Bible or a quote in a medical journal without first understanding the surrounding context.

Islam puts a large emphasis on treating the spiritual and physical together to create optimum health. This is why Islam prescribes prayer with medicine and food with lifestyle changes. Islam promotes attaining a physical health that is only possible through congruent spiritual, psychological, and mindful practice. Together, this unity comprises a holistic approach to health.

If we ignore this unity, 'treating the cause' can be a challenge for us. We are so used to blaming the organs, genes, and body parts for our aches and pains that when we fail to consider the interrelationship between the different aspects of our health, we cannot recognise the true root of the problem.

When I tell my patients we need to explore the causes around their conditions, they are unable to recognise what the causes could be. They have never considered the other parts of the elephant and have only ever viewed their symptoms in isolation from the rest of the body. The cause is always multifactorial. I have never come across a disease that is triggered by just one thing. Thus, there is no one drug that fits all, no magical pill that fixes everything. Even if the additional causes comprise only a small portion of the overarching problem, it is essential to delineate them so treatment can be wholly effective. Without considering every slice of the pie, we get an incomplete and linear view of the disease.

A growing body of research speaks to how the health of the sperm, egg, and mother – relative to her quality of life regarding diet, exercise, stress, rest, and supplements – have a very important role to play in the development of offspring. This is called epigenetics. In 2005, the Environmental Working Group (EWG) conducted a study into the pollution of newborns through analysis of umbilical cord blood. They discovered a total of 287 chemicals within the umbilical cords that were tested, of which 180 were known carcinogens, while the remaining chemicals were toxins to the brain and nervous system or causes of birth defects.[38] In a society that pumps tens of thousands of unregulated or, I should say, under-regulated chemicals into the environment, it is no wonder that cancer rates continue to increase.

In linear culture, the cancer and disease narrative goes something like this: "Everything has chemicals in it, so there is nothing you can do about it," and, "Just trust conventional treatments because there are no alternatives." Both points stem from the truth. There really *are* chemicals in everything, and there really *isn't* a cure for cancer because, the truth is, cancer has no one cause. However, there are other questions we should be asking.

Why don't we have any knowledge about how we can reduce chemicals in our own homes? Why doesn't anyone talk about detoxing the body? What are the other parts of the elephant? With the millions we invest in finding a drug treatment for cancer, why don't we invest more in preventing cancer? Why is there such an oxymoron in our linear approach, so much so that we use products that could potentially cause cancer, such as underarm deodorants laced with known carcinogens, to bring awareness to the disease?

A few years ago, a young couple who had gone through IVF (in vitro fertilisation) twice and had no success falling pregnant came to see me.

The man had no sperm. They even went to the extent of cutting open his scrotum to see whether any sperm was stuck inside that could be used for IVF or ICSI (intracytoplasmic sperm injection) but found nothing. It was mind-blowing to me. Why wasn't this 30-year-old man producing sperm? Was it a lack of nutrition? Too much radiation? Did he have an autoimmune disease? I needed to uncover the driving factor to understand if he had any hope at all of becoming a father one day.

As I talked with the couple, I discovered that the man worked in the steel business. In fact, he worked for a company that made copper pipes. I tested his hair sample for heavy metals, and, lo and behold, his copper levels were through the roof!

As you may or may not know, contraception comes in various forms. And what is one of these forms? The copper IUD (intrauterine device). Why is copper used in this form of contraception? Because it is a spermicide. Potentially, this man's contact with copper had rendered him infertile, possibly reducing his sperm production to nil because of the toxic exposure. His body had been systematically poisoned with copper to such an extent that it was either not producing any sperm, or it was producing very little and killing it off before it had an opportunity to fertilise the egg or even fully mature. At least, this was my take on it as a holistic functional medicine practitioner.

While some literature discusses the negative effects that a surplus of copper can have on the male reproductive system, not enough research has been conducted to establish a definitive connection.[39] However, when I look at a patient's problem from a holistic perspective, I am not looking for a definitive connection. I am trying to find things that stand out as potential drivers of the overarching condition. When I was told about his work with copper, it seemed clear that it could have an impact on his fertility.

This does not mean that everyone who works with copper will become infertile. That is kind of like saying, "Everyone who smokes will get lung cancer," or, "Everyone who deals with mercury will develop mercury poisoning." However, for this particular man, due to certain single nucleotide polymorphisms (SNPs) in his liver, the decreased ability of his liver to detox heavy metals, and other health challenges he bore, his elevated copper levels were detrimental to his fertility. Like the straw that broke the camel's back, his copper toxicity was the main driver but was also just one factor among a myriad of others that contributed to the total pie of causes.

We had to cleanse the body of copper, a process that would take one full year. However, the problem was that for eight hours per day, five days per week, the man was exposed to the very toxin that was preventing him from producing sperm – or was killing the sperm before it was manufactured enough to move into the ejaculatory system. There was a clear and concise connection. In this very rare circumstance, I suggested that the man change jobs, which was something I would *never* normally do. Because we checked his liver for SNPs and discovered that he had a genetic weakness in the heavy metal detox pathways, we had to reduce exposure if we wanted to get real results.

The downside to this story is that though we started the copper detox program, the couple cancelled their next appointment. They decided to go overseas and try IVF for a third time, even though the man had no sperm. The couple did not want to commit to a year-long detoxification process. Fast forward four years, and the couple still have not been able to conceive. This is the sad reality for many of us.

When something is not mainstream, it often gets dismissed or left in the dark. The truth is that often such ideas represent forward thinking. This kind of thinking is cutting-edge, but it also goes against the mainstream narrative and if it is not mainstream, people struggle to accept it. I urge you to consider alternative treatments. We may all have the same anatomy, but our bodily responses that create disease can vary immensely. That is why we functional medical practitioners do not see every man and woman who suffer the same ailments as having the same driving factors. We look into each case on an individual and unique level, working to understand the psychological and contextual underpinnings of every patient.

For too long, we have allowed an institutionalised medical system to pull apart our organs and treat our bodies like machines, throwing out a piece when it does not work, as opposed to treating the cause of illness. As a result, we have created a space where people have more cancers and autoimmune illnesses than ever before, and our children are suffering from more ailments today than any child did 60 years ago.[40] We must collectively look inward to discover how we can better our wellbeing and actively seek answers to our own health questions.

So, which parts of the elephant had you seen, and which parts were you blind to?

CHAPTER THREE

CONNECTING HEALTH AND THE MIND

In Islam, we are guided to be hopeful and optimistic and to put our trust in God. Though this is the cornerstone of our religion, it is not without caveat. When we place our trust in God, we must also 'tie our camel'.

Uh, what…? Let me explain.

By placing our trust in Allah, we are not void of free will and personal responsibility. Yes, we must have hope and faith in our lord to guide, protect, and show us the way through life, but we also have the ability to create our own destiny through positive action. In fact, in the Qur'an, it is noted that the only thing a Muslim *cannot* change is her or his birth and death. This concept is not unique to Islam and applies even if you are not religious. How often do you think that because of circumstances beyond your control, you cannot change your destiny? After all, as a conscious human, your responsibility lies in the journey, not the end result. The end result is for Him to decree. However, the journey to the end result is what we are responsible for. For everything that is outside our control, there is a list of things that are not. We each have the power to mould our own lives, despite the hand of cards we are dealt. After all, it is not what happens to us that matters most. Instead, how we deal with and respond – rather than react – to what happens to us is paramount.

Destiny, fate, or God – whatever you believe in – does not dish out every problem in our lives. Much of our suffering comes from our own action, or inaction. This can be a hard pill to swallow. In surah Ar-Ra'd of the Qur'an verse 11, Allah says, "We will not change the condition of a people until they change what is within themselves." This alone is enough for any conscious believer to acknowledge that through free will and responsibility much is left to us to steer and create our own destiny in relation to many things in life.

Take gastrointestinal problems, for example. Almost everyone can relate to experiencing some form of gut issue in their lives. Perhaps we were born with the gene that predisposes us to an illness, or perhaps we were not. Whether the gene is readily turned on or not, when we live a high-stress lifestyle, make poor diet choices, and experience excess exposure to chemicals, we increase the likelihood of developing health problems or exacerbating our pre-existing conditions. As I like to put it: if the gene is the gun, the environment is the trigger. Without pulling the trigger, the bullet cannot reach its destination. Similarly, without environmental exposure to provoke certain genes to turn on, you may live life with many potential genes in your genome that remain switched off or continue to turn on.

For example, my husband has hay fever, and I do not. We have three children together, a boy and two girls. If everything were genetics alone, then, theoretically, one of the two children would suffer from hay fever. But they do not. Now, this does not necessarily mean that they will never experience these problems. It is possible that those genes have been passed down but are not switched on *at the moment.* 'At the moment' is a very important phrase here because an inactive gene now does not mean an inactive gene forever. Let me explain further.

If my children pursued an unhealthy lifestyle by eating lots of processed foods, therefore, contributing to poor gut function and a plethora of immune issues, and if they were not getting enough exercise, sleep, and managing their stress levels, they would have created conditions for certain genes to switch on. In contrast, if they chose to pursue life consciously, eating organic wholefoods, getting adequate rest, detoxing, exercising, and managing their breath, they may not have that gene turned on during their time on this earth plane. Let us discuss exercise in more detail. Research suggests that exercising can keep certain genes switched off and contribute to turning on beneficial genes.[41] None of this is new information. There is ample literature discussing how environmental factors can contribute to evolving gene expression, for better or worse.[42]

Our genes are not our destiny. Blaming genes for bad health is really creating a scapegoat for the tremendous responsibility and control we have over our health. For example, it is so much easier to look at it like this: you have high cholesterol because your dad has high cholesterol. You may neglect to consider that you also have the same environment as your father: a sedentary lifestyle, a high-stress life, a diet high in refined carbohydrates and animal products.

There is a lot we can do to prevent disease while our babies are in the womb or even before that, during preconception. This is called epigenetics, which is "the study of changes in organisms caused by modification of gene expression rather than alteration of the genetic code itself."[43] Therefore, the choices I make as a conscious parent – elongating breastfeeding, drinking filtered water, supplementing during breastfeeding, eating organic produce, reducing exposure to toxicity in the home

– decrease the risk associated with epigenetic presentation of disease. This is what I referred to earlier as 'free will and responsibility'.

Islamically, in fact, you are not responsible for a sin you have committed if you were unaware of it being a sin in the first place. Our job as parents is not to guilt trip ourselves for making poor choices for our children or ourselves but once we know it was a poor choice, to proactively change is the goal. By the end of this book, God willing, you will have the knowledge you need, and the responsibility to use it well will be yours.

I also want to acknowledge that although doing all the right things can reduce the risk of illness and disease, if it is God's decree, it will still occur. However, it is rare to hear that someone had an illness and a perfectly healthy lifestyle versus the more common example of someone who had an illness and many areas to correct in their diet and lifestyle choices.

Our job, so to speak, is to tie the camel and submit to the will of God at the same time. If illness comes to you and you do your best regarding free will and responsibility, then there is nothing to worry about. However, we know as Muslims that on the day of resurrection, not us but our body parts will speak on our behalf in relation to what we did with them. In this case, you are responsible for everything you have conscious control over that may have contributed to your presenting health condition and symptoms.

The Mind-Body Connection

It is no secret that our mind creates our reality. Think about it. How often do your thoughts impact your experiences?

Consider the law of attraction: the idea that by thinking positive thoughts, positive experiences will be brought into your life. The same goes for negative thoughts, which, when focused on, bring about negative experiences.

Let me give you some examples. You buy a car. Now, up until today, you cannot really recollect seeing this make and model on the road. However, now that you own this particular car, you see them *everywhere*. That is the law of attraction in action. Your brain makes you consciously aware of something that was previously in the subconscious that you have now coded your mind to focus on. The cars were always there, but it was not an important piece of information before you bought one, so your mind never alerted you to it.

Now, imagine that you have had a bad day. First, your car stopped working; then you lost your car keys, could not get into the house, and got news that your friend was in hospital. You might think it was all coincidence, but everything is vibration and energy. The more we focus on negative things in life, the more we attract them. Perhaps this is one of the reasons why Islam asks us to set out intention prior to every prayer we intend. This is not new-age gibberish for us; this was set in stone 1400 years ago, so to speak. We are to live life through consciousness, through intention, and through bringing awareness of every single thing we do to our conscious minds. We are spiritual beings manifesting in a three-dimensional body; therefore, there is a spiritual reality to us. Not everything that occurs is the result of our five senses. There is more to us and this earth plane than that.

This concept can be very triggering. For some people, the idea that their misfortune could be 'their fault' is quite confrontational, especially when we so comfortably live in a state of victimhood and denial. Now, I am not here to play the blame game. There are things in everybody's lives that they are not responsible for nor had any part in bringing to fruition. What I am saying is that our attitude has the power to influence what comes our way and how we choose to experience it. It is not what happens to you that dictates your life; it is your perception of it. Realizing this is very empowering.

Imagine that you know a volatile and abusive alcoholic. He has two sons. One of the sons ends up being exactly like his father. He becomes an alcoholic, gets married, and abuses his children. The other son chooses a different path. He excels in work and is a very conscious and caring father.

You ask the first son, "Why did you end up being an alcoholic?" He says, "How can I not be? My dad was my example." Then you ask the other son, "How did you not become an alcoholic and instead are so kind and successful?" He says, "How can I not? Look at my father." What is the difference between the two sons? Their perception and attitude, which has ultimately affected their life experiences.

Now, how does this all translate when it comes to our health?

It is no secret that the brain impacts the physical being. There is no such thing as a healthy body if the mind is not healthy too, and vice versa. Ninety percent of hormones, such as serotonin and melatonin, are in fact made in the small intestine, not in the brain, which means what we eat actually controls how we feel.[44] Is that not an important point to remember when we consider how and why Islamic medicine plays such a crucial role in preventing illness and maintaining health? We now scientifically acknowledge that food is a critical driver for our mental health.

Serotonin is in fact the hormone that makes you feel happy, and melatonin is the antioxidant hormone that helps us fall asleep. The very process of falling asleep due to high levels of this hormone means that, during sleep, we can gear towards the healing we were unable to do during the day while the body was busy keeping up with other things. Without serotonin, we cannot even make melatonin, meaning that sometimes poor sleep is not the main contributor to poor mood. It is in fact the other way around: poor serotonin levels mean that a depressed or stressed person cannot get good sleep because they need ample amounts of this hormone to make melatonin.

Let us look at how our mental health affects our physical wellness. Positive thoughts generate oxytocin and serotonin. Yes, thoughts can affect the neuroplasticity of the brain.

Looking at the prefrontal cortex, when happy thoughts occur, brain growth takes place through the reinforcement and generation of new synapses. The prefrontal cortex is where all mind/brain functions conjugate and are dispersed to various parts of the brain or transmitted to other parts of the body. The prefrontal cortex is the switching station that regulates the signals from neurons and allows us to reflect and think about what we are currently doing. It allows us to control our emotions through our deep limbic brain. Since it allows us to focus, the prefrontal cortex also gives us time for metacognition: being aware of our own thought processes.

Visualisation for Good Health

Similar to the law of attraction, visualisation can be a handy tool to help attract what you want in life. When you focus on achieving specific goals, your brain subconsciously produces ideas that help you reach that goal. Regularly visualising your objectives also keeps you motivated to achieve them, as they remain at the forefront of your mind.

For example, about eight years ago, I made a vision board for all my goals. To be honest, it was quite superficial: a car, a nice house, and other rather superficial goals. After about three months of staring at that board every day – not even consciously, just staring at it because it was in the room where I consulted – I ended up purchasing a new car. What's more, it was the same car from the photo on my vision board: a Porsche Boxster. It was the exact same model, colour, everything. I didn't even have a conscious recognition of cutting out and sticking that particular car. This method works the same way when it comes to our health goals.

Visualisation is, in essence, the act of seeing with your mind prior to something manifesting on a physical plane. So, you are seeing it with your mind before you see it with your eyes. We live in a vibrational universe. This is practically proven now and literally means that nothing around us is solid. It is empty space, coming in and out of existence from another dimension. Let us delve in a little bit more.

In Islam, one of God's names and attributes is Al Kaliq, which means 'the creator', but it does not mean that he created the Universe and then gained that name. That is, he didn't become the creator after he created the Universe. Al Kaliq actually means "the one who is constantly creating and bringing into existence." So, during every millisecond of our existence on this earth plane, Allah is creating. He is constantly bringing into existence the environment in which we live, our bodies, and everything we consider to be 'matter'. Through quantum physics, science has finally begun to entertain the idea that we are in fact energy as much as we are 'solid mass'. We are constantly vibrating and coming in and out of existence, and that, in essence, is the law of attraction. Creation is constantly occurring and will continue to occur until the horn is blown, so to speak.

Consider Salatul Istikhara, one of our prayers: the prayer of seeking counsel. Fourteen hundred years ago, we were given a prayer to guide us to the best result regarding an idea or embarking on something. We are taught that we set the intention. We pray; we *focus* on the idea and if Allah wills that prayer, the dream or aspiration becomes a reality. So, we are focusing on the intention of what we want, and we are using our emotional selves to experience it, which attracts the vibrational pull.

In tasawwuf (Islamic mysticism), we are taught to negate any negative beliefs by focusing on positive thoughts so we are less affected by the whispers and satanic and animalistic desires that the ego and physical self come with.

I could go on and on, but it is time to move on to the next topic.

How to Change Your Mindset Around Food

Ninety-nine percent of the time, the women I work with have a very deep emotional connection to food. Because they have been told to suppress their emotions, to put others before themselves, to compromise, to be the 'perfect' woman, wife, and mother, they have grown up unable to express their true selves. Generally, until we have a chat, they have no awareness of the fact that they are who they are due to cultural moulding, and they are yet to genuinely and authentically shine in their own light. They make themselves small and mould their identities to 'fit in' out of fear of judgement. So, to fill this emotional void, they turn to food. They think, "This will make me feel good because I have nothing else that will." And it does, even if temporarily.

Cheese is a good example of a food that provides an extra level of comfort and can boost our moods. A study that aimed to discover which foods are the most addictive found cheese to be almost as problematic as cake and soda.[45] Some believe that casein, the primary protein found in dairy, produces an opiate-like effect in the body and the brain. Simply put, cheese may be acting just like a drug! No wonder so many of us find it addictive. The truth is that years ago when I experimented with veganism, cheese was definitely one of the hardest things to let go of, and now I know why. Ali, the son-in-law and cousin of our prophet, Muhammad (peace be upon them both), is believed to have said, "Do not make your stomachs graveyards of animals." Because cheese is the by-product of an animal, an excretion, a discharge, we acknowledge the importance of keeping foods such as cheese in the list of those we should not consume too often.

So, where does that put milk chocolate or any other sweet food made with dairy? Now, we know that the emotional relationship to food is more than just a psychological connection, but also a biochemical reality.

As a practitioner, I can give my clients the best diet, supplements, and lifestyle advice but until their mindsets change, the physical body will stay the same. Even if someone follows the health advice to a tee, an unfit mindset will hinder their progress. When the client has another fight with their husband, disconnects from their authentic self, submits to judgement and self-loathing, develops hate for their appearance, focuses on someone else's negative comments about them, does not get enough sleep, or when some other issue arises, guess what they turn to for emotional support? Food!

As long as food is a source of emotional comfort, we will forever breed disease. Abu Huraira, a friend of the Prophet (PBUH), narrates: "The family of Muhammad did not eat their fill for three successive days till he died."[46] This statement and others were not just passed on to acknowledge hunger or fasting – on the contrary. They acknowledge the devastating effects that overconsuming food has on our physical and mental health.

When we constantly eat unhealthy foods, in amounts and at times that we should not, we put a huge strain on the body. The liver works harder;

the stomach produces extra acid, and the body requires more sleep to recuperate, as all energy is taxed by the digestive system. Thus, less is left for other systems of the body to heal. Then the bowels go into overdrive, trying to expel the excess toxic load. Suddenly, your physical energy is expended cleaning out toxins rather than recuperating and rejuvenating the body.

No one can come into true and complete physical health without also addressing their mental health. Why? Because someone who does not love themselves enough to make a psychological change is not ready for a physical transformation. Any change outside of this can only ever be temporary. Have you watched *The Biggest Loser*? Have you noticed that the vast majority of the contestants always end up regaining the weight they lose within a handful of years? Why? Because a change that does not address the mind and trauma that created the habit and the poor relationship with food can only ever be short-lasting and is doomed to resurface when the time is right.

This may be why God says that intentions are just as important as actions. Once we come into a state of awareness of our emotional health, make the intention, and pray for our overall healing, God's help will be near, as promised in the Qur'an through a Sahih Hadith via a Muslim narration:

> Whoever comes with a good deed will have the reward of ten like it and even more. Whoever comes with an evil deed will be recompensed for one evil deed like it or he will be forgiven. Whoever draws close to Me by the length of a hand, I will draw close to him by the length of an arm. Whoever draws close to Me by the length of an arm, I will draw close to him by the length of a fathom. Whoever comes to Me walking, I will come to him running. Whoever meets Me with enough sins to fill the earth, not associating any partners with Me, I will meet him with as much forgiveness.

On the flip side, experiencing a significant health scare is sometimes enough to shock a person into a new mindset. Although I do not think it should take tragedy or illness to make a health change, it *can* work. If someone experiences a heart attack, stroke, or major hospitalisation, it is quite common for that person to actively make modifications to their lifestyle. This is because their mindset says, *If I keep doing this, I'm going to die early*, or, *I'm going to live the rest of my life diseased*. When the penny drops, they start to make essential changes that inevitably provoke a lifelong transformation. Is this the best way to change? Probably not.

Initiating healthy lifestyle changes through conscious awareness in the absence of illness or disease may be better. The very awareness of the connection between the body and soul and how the two work hand in hand comes from the truth that we are spiritual beings manifesting in a three-dimensional body. If we were all spirit, the body would have no weight. In contrast, if we were all focused on the body, then the spirit would have no weight, and, sad to say, some of us are like this. A person with a lack of consciousness resembles other mammals that have no conscious awareness, and choices are made based on the needs of the physical body only. There are no spiritual needs for an animal, as it does not carry a spirit in the way a human being does. This is why when we focus only on our physical body, we are effectively aiding the animalistic side of our creation.

Physics and the Spiritual Body

Ever heard of $E = mc^2$? It is Einstein's famous equation for how energy is in fact the mass of an object times the speed of light squared. Why am I raising this when I am talking about food and mental health? Because the human has both a spiritual and physical truth to him. Because man can become more energy or more mass depending on what he does with himself.

E is energy; m is mass, and c is the speed of light, which does not change. So, Einstein is saying that if the speed of light does not change and if something reaches the speed of light, then mass can turn into energy, and energy can turn into mass. If I throw a brick at someone, that brick will only reach where I aim it because it is a solid object. However, if I shine a light on someone, the light will shine on many things at the same time because it is not a solid mass.

In one experiment, researchers have a plank of wood with two holes in it. They use a gun to shoot a bullet at the plank, and the bullet exits through one of the holes. As solid mass, the bullet cannot possibly exit at more than one location. However, when researchers try the same experiment with water, squirting it at the plank, they find that the liquid travels through both holes because it is not a solid mass.

Next, they try the same experiment with an electron gun. When researchers shoot electrons at the plank, the particles go through both holes at the same time, behaving not as an object with mass but as one with waves, like a light or laser.

Researchers then attempt to measure why electrons – which should behave as solid mass – are acting like energy. So, they add a device to monitor the behaviour of the electrons and repeat the experiment. However, the electrons start behaving as solid mass, only travelling through one hole at a time. The simple act of observing the experiment changes the outcome.

Let us look at this from an Islamic perspective. We understand that when we approach something below its atomic mass, the object changes from presenting as mass and reverts to acting like a wave. It changes from tangible – a solid object – to something intangible, like light or sound.

For example, if I only feed my physical body, I may be physically strong and muscular, but I will also develop other mass-like qualities, such as a sole desire for the tangible world, for money and other items of finite value, for all that is superficial and physical in its nature. At the same time, my spirit is trapped in a spiritually void prison. In contrast, if I neglect to feed my physical body and invest only in feeding my spiritual body, my spirit will overpower my physical mass, and I will become more intangible, more like a light or wavelength.

Have you heard the story of Somuncu Baba, a 17th century scholar who dedicated his life to Islam? He was once upon a time seen coming out of three separate doors of the same mosque at the same time. He achieved this through the very equation Einstein was labelled a genius for discovering. Because Somuncu Baba's spiritual body was so well-nourished, his physical body had become less like mass and more like light or sound.

When we instead feed our physical body and neglect the spiritual, we become more mass than spirit. This is mostly the state of our current world, which lacks the spiritual compass and contains more mass than spirit. And, lo and behold, we have a plethora of man-made problems – heightened levels of depression, anxiety, and disconnection – that are mostly associated with not filling our spiritual voids with the correct alignment. We exist in a world full of unused human potential that is wasted when it is held at the animal level.

Three Facets of an Unshakable Mindset

1. AWARENESS

Awareness is the first port of call when attempting to look at anything in its wholeness, and this of course applies to food. What we do not know, we really do not know; therefore, where there is no awareness, there really is no awareness.

When we just see food as something that satiates our taste buds, enters one hole and exits another, we lack awareness of how it contributes to our thought processes, our physical wellness, our mental wellness, and our telomeres, thus, either shortening or elongating our lives. Food affects every aspect of every single cell in our bodies. Once we become aware, the next step is to learn which foods are beneficial for what, which foods cause problems in the body, what these problems are, and how to deal with junk and processed foods in the 21st century as people navigating through food choice chaos. Then what in heaven should we eat?!

Let us switch the discussion to eczema. The typical treatment for eczema is cortisone, as it can reduce the redness and itchiness of the skin, reducing the appearance of the eczema. But eczema generally does not disappear just like that. When we use cortisone, we simply suppress the issue short-term. It does not treat the underlying problem, meaning that the steroid may need to be used on and off forever. The treatment definitely gives the patient some relief from the constant discomfort, which is no doubt a godsend, but, really, we are only suppressing a symptom. If the eczema does heal, it is not because of the cortisone but due to the immune system doing the work necessary to restore the body to homeostasis.

Now, how does that tie in with the concept of awareness?

People often treat eczema with corticosteroids because they are unaware of other treatment options, or, while they assume alternatives exist, they have a sense of urgency and do not want to lose time investigating other treatments. There are many underlying causes of eczema that we, as functional medicine practitioners, treat holistically. Too often, taking children off foods that their immune system and gut do not tolerate, healing the lining of the gut, and fixing up their nutritional deficiencies may allow them to not only come off cortisone, but also to heal from their eczema. Each case is, of course, individual in its cause.

A one-year-old boy came to me with blood oozing from his face because of how often he itched himself due to his eczema. He was on cortisone; however, at this stage, he was not responding to the cortisone, the bleach baths, or any other conventional medicine treatments. His mum was clearly at her wits' end, crying due to being completely emotionally overwhelmed by the constant lectures she received from people who saw the state of her son's face and assumed she was not doing enough. However, she was doing everything she had awareness of and once she had awareness of the potential of seeing a health practitioner, she came to me.

Within three months, the boy's eczema was 70 percent better, and he was off his cortisone drugs. By month five, he was 99 percent clear of any eczema symptoms as well as all others, including intolerance to some foods and poor gut motility (constipation). Due to constant itching and bleeding, his sleep quality had been poor, which made him an angry and introverted child. Healing his eczema restored his quality of sleep, thus, improving his overall temperament and mood. I will never forget his face when he first came to my clinic and when we completed the healing program and we were ready to part ways. Both versions – before and after treatment – are forever framed in my mind.

Food can cause *countless* health issues, but, due to a lack of awareness, we rarely stop to consider that what we are ingesting might be the root of these problems. Without this awareness, we are less likely to change our mindsets around the food that causes us harm and, therefore, less likely to heal from health challenges that those very food, lifestyle, and environmental choices create.

2. HEALING TRAUMA

Trauma has a big role to play in a person's mindset toward food. For many of us, food is a lot more than just the sustenance we need to survive. It is comfort, support, happiness, and relief. Often, we turn to food to fill voids in other areas of our lives. This generally results in not only *eating* poor foods but *overeating* them.

Ibn Qayyim was a theologian of the 11th century. In his book, *Healing with the Medicine of the Prophet*, he writes largely on prophetic and preventative medicine, claiming that many illnesses occur due to our consumption of food before our initial meal has been digested.[47] In the current day and age, this is one of the reasons why fasting is so famous and why there is so much literature on how it heals the body from many illnesses. The very abstinence of food is healing, not the overconsumption of it. I will speak more on this in chapter seven, which discusses fasting in depth.

We have become tremendously attached to overeating as a form of emotional lullaby, and herein lies many of our health challenges. To detach ourselves from emotional eating, we must first acknowledge and understand where that attachment comes from. We must be aware that we are not eating only because we are hungry but also because we are happy, sad, anxious, numbing our depression, or socialising, alongside many other reasons that should not relate to food. It is up to us to work through this response with self-compassion and self-love.

Here is a classic example of this: a client comes to me and says, "I've been on a diet for years, but I'm always gaining weight back." In this client's case, the first questions they need to ask themselves are, *What is the mental pattern that keeps creating the same physical reality that I am trying to detach myself from? Why do I keep returning to unhealthy eating habits? What is it about consistent exercise that I just can't cope with?*

The reason could be a litany of things: a stressful home life, an unfulfilling career, poor body image – the list goes on. It is up to the client to identify and work through whatever part of her life is causing the blockage. Nine times out of ten, it all boils down to a lack of self-love. This shortage of love not only makes it harder for us to stick to long-term goals that benefit us, but it also leaves us reluctant to seek support and invest in our own health and happiness.

For example, a lot of people refuse to see a naturopath, coach, personal trainer, nutritionist, or psychologist. They believe it is "too expensive," which is completely justified. Life *is* expensive and if you are struggling to make ends meet, these services are probably not at the top of your priority list. However, if you still go out and spend $80 on a lipstick and $300 on a pair of shoes, even though you already have a few perfectly fine pairs at home, then the reason is not that you cannot afford a naturopath; it is that you do not think your health and happiness are worth the investment.

In our high-paced modern society, we consider anything that takes more than a couple of minutes to be unfeasible, and we settle for quick fixes. We want answers, and we want them now! How do we get those immediate answers? Through an emotional connection to food. The minute we ingest it, we send certain signals to the brain that activate happiness. It happens quickly, which is why food is such an addictive drug. The belief that we cannot afford to invest in ourselves in a meaningful way stems from a direct lack of self-worth and not wanting to invest in anything that takes time – because we are so impatient.

Let me give you a personal example. My mum and I had this conversation about a year ago, and she said something profound. I said to her, "Mum, you need to book your physiotherapist more consistently. You've got time, you've got money, you've got energy, you've got a car, you've got all the resources."

"But it's too expensive," she said.

Now, her physiotherapy only costs $50 per session; therefore, she can comfortably pay for it. But in her mind, she would rather spend it on her grandchildren, shopping for the house, or buying ingredients to make a nice dessert for the family. Why? Because that's what drives her sense of self-worth and makes her feel empowered. She gets her self-worth from doing things for others, like many of us who are brainwashed by the cultural normality of giving to everyone else but ourselves. Society gives us a gold medal for acting this way and, because we are so void of self-love, we require that reward to keep going.

We think our religion tells us to do more and give more – but does it really? If that is the case, why is the obligatory charity for a Muslim only 2.5 percent of your wealth? You keep 97.5 percent and give only a tiny portion. If it is religion and not culture that demands doing more for others, why does a Hadith imply otherwise? A woman comes to the Prophet (PBUH) to complain that her husband is neglecting her because he is spending long nights praying. The Prophet's response to her is that he prays, but he spends time with his women too; he fasts, but he also consumes foods; he does night prayers, but also spends night-time in a state of sleep.

These are all beautiful examples that highlight the importance of moderation as the actual alignment stick of our religion and, thus, our lifestyle as Islam. Often, many of us – whether we follow the path of atheism, Christianity, Judaism, or anything else – have cultural conditioning embedded in our values. We hold these tainted values dear, as though they come from religion, but they do not, and the enmeshment of religion and culture can certainly become an issue.

Often, when we need to invest in ourselves but neglect to do so, it is not always that we do not have the money; it is that we do not think our money is worth being spent in that particular area. This behaviour is common in a lot of us, especially when our self-worth comes from external factors. We are willing to spend money sending our kids to extracurricular activities because this satiates the ego. People will say that so and so sends their kids to ballet or taekwondo or whatever the activity is. What a wonderful mother/father/caretaker they are! We seek to fill that self-love cup that would otherwise be empty.

Similarly, we may be happy to buy our friends dinner but refuse to fork out the extra cash for our own healthy meal plans. If we genuinely dig deep and self-reflect, we will see that what we do for others is driven by how it makes us feel. Again, we fill the void of self-love by doing for others what we generally think is not worth doing for ourselves. Not only do we fill our emotional void, but we also stay distracted and safe from any need for inner change and healing. We often think that the only way we will ever be satiated with happiness is if we keep doing things for others because that is what drives our sense of self-worth. When we feel unworthy, spending money on our own wellbeing seems like a waste because, after all, we are not worthy. We believe that investing in ourselves is not going to give us that feeling of happiness and contentment we get from doing things for others.

In the following chapter, we will delve more deeply into food and trauma. For now, it is important to note that our behaviour and mindset around food is influenced by pain. Healing this pain will heal the mindset and when the mindset is healed, change and positive metamorphosis occurs. When we see a butterfly struggling to escape its cocoon, we instinctively want to help it, so we decide to break the cocoon to set the insect free. Although this seems like a beneficial act, it is completely to the contrary. If we assist the butterfly, it misses out on developing the muscles needed to fly; therefore, it will die. In the same way, the only way to liberate is through pain. To paraphrase Rumi, the pain is where the healing enters. If we live our lives in fear of pain, healing will never occur.

3. KNOWLEDGE AND RESOURCES

We are unable to make change without first acquiring the knowledge and resources needed to get us on the right track.

For example, let us say you have a gluten sensitivity and go to the supermarket to buy some bread. You pick up the first loaf you see and think, *Yep, that says gluten-free – great,* and you pop it in the trolley. However, what you did not see was the long list of chemicals that comprised the ingredients. You lacked this knowledge and, therefore, only focused on the one thing: whether gluten was present or not. Just like the blind men, you only saw one part of the elephant and assumed it was the whole thing. Sometimes products labelled 'gluten-free' still contain wheat; however, the gluten component may have been chemically removed from the bread. Sometimes, the chemicals used may be more detrimental to our health than the gluten itself.

Knowledge and resources are very important for changing a person's mindset around health and food. Perhaps this is why the first verse revealed to man by God in the Qur'an was IQRA, which translates to 'read'. The importance of learning and growth from cradle to grave, especially for Muslims, can only ever be understated.

People often say, "I know I get bloated when I have dairy, but I love cheese and don't know what else to eat." Because they do not have the appropriate knowledge or resources, they do not know what to try that will taste equally as good but will not harm their health. On top of this, they do not know where to find the right food or how much it should cost. Therefore, their lack of knowledge drives them away from making a change. However, you do not have to know everything; you just need to know where to look. I am no Islamic scholar, but the Qur'an is written in a way that all laymen can understand, so for me it is about knowing where to look and using my brain to critically and constructively evaluate the information in front of me until it either strengthens my conviction or breaks it.

As a naturopath, my job is to help set the foundation for my clients' optimum health. I have the knowledge and resources, and it is my responsibility to share these with my clients, which I do. However, if someone does not do the work themselves, my input will be largely futile. You know the proverb, "You can lead a horse to water, but you can't make him drink." That is exactly what it is like.

I do not spoonfeed my clients. I do not want to create co-dependency. I want my clients to have the autonomy, authority, and power to exist in my absence – to be independent. Achieving independence is massively challenging for anyone in our culture because we grow up in families who are enmeshed emotionally, who lack boundaries, and who are co-dependent. Even today, as a parent, I suffer from emotional co-dependency with my children, and I know this is an area I need to work on, so I do. I first acknowledge that the challenge is preventing me from becoming the best version of myself. I then make my intention, put my trust in God, and look proactively for human and non-human resources to help me. After all, that is all we can do, and Allah is the one who heals and turns hearts. We are only looking to find catalysts. He is the one who says "be," and it is.

If a client is in need of knowledge, I discuss it with them during consultation. Then, I usually give them two websites that I love and trust, saying, "Off you go, go and do some research." In the case of a specific product – for example, bread – I might suggest a type but encourage the client to use trial and error to find one that fits them: "If you don't like this, try one with buckwheat. If you don't like buckwheat, try one with quinoa. If you don't like that, try one with rice."

Whether or not you engage a naturopath, you have a responsibility to gain knowledge and resources if you want to change your mindset around food. No one else is going to do it for you. It might sound harsh, but there is nobody who will ever care about your health as much as you do – because you live in your body. Your spirit resides there, and the level of comfort and discomfort you feel each and every day is specific and personal to you. Start by trawling the internet, picking up some books, and seeking professional advice. Once you begin to understand exactly what you are putting in your body, you will be surprised how quickly your mindset around food changes. You will slowly acknowledge that in order to consciously connect with the Creator, we must always be in a state of conscious living and consumption, which is the motto that helped me write this book.

Addiction

When it comes to acknowledging addiction, we are not just talking about alcohol and drugs. We are talking about addiction to food, addiction to sex, addiction to superficiality, addiction to shopping, addiction to social media, addiction to anything that numbs our souls and our pain, anything that allows us to avoid feeling pain and turning inwards. Why do we do this? Because we know that this society has long ago embedded into our subconscious that pain sucks; pain is horrible, and no one should ever feel it. Addiction is anything that is done or dosed more than necessary. When I talk about addiction, I want you to understand that it is a wide umbrella. All addiction matters.

Addiction looks different to everyone. It is not reserved for the poor or the weak or the less fortunate. We all have addictions, and the more readily we accept this, the more able we will be to remove the stigma of addiction and heal ourselves and each other.

Part of the reason why I wanted to write this book was to show you that *everyone* has their struggles. I am not some perfect person sitting in an ivory tower, claiming to hold all the answers. I am still learning! I have my own flaws, my own demons to face (in the next chapter, I will share more of this with you). In saying that, there are some problems that I have not come up against, and I will never claim to have first-hand experience combatting those issues in my own life. I am sharing my experiences not as an expert per se but as a human navigating this three-dimensional experience called life, using the Qur'an as my compass for direction and alignment.

For now, I would like to share my own addiction that is very much still a work in progress.

I think we can all agree that buying creams for your skin or balms for your lips is pretty harmless. Of course, we can go out and spend money on products that make our lashes longer and brows darker. But when does this go too far? When does this need to look 'perfect' border on addiction? Is it when we spend every pay cheque filling our faces with botox and filler? Or is it when we become so uncomfortable in our own skin that we cannot take a photo without filtering our faces until they are almost unrecognisable?

I am not immune to addiction. I am at risk of experiencing all these desires, just like everyone else. The only thing that makes me different is that I have awareness of my actions and addiction, which means I can turn my knowledge into action. I know it is very scary to change, to acknowledge your own shadows and demons, but it is also the only way out. There is no other detour; there is no other shortcut. You have to drive along that highway if you want to truly heal.

My biggest addiction is doing anything that helps me dissociate. Let me explain. When I am confronted with something that makes me feel big feelings, ones I am not sure how to – or too scared to – process, I disconnect; I avoid; I switch off. Sometimes this translates to me being the workaholic mum. Other times, if it is my inner child that needs healing, the healing is too scary, so I take away from myself and oversaturate my children with time and energy. Other times, I bury my sorrows in hours of housework or reading – whatever works for me at that stage to disconnect from those thoughts and feelings.

This is all learned behaviour. I remember as a child having experiences where my very own caretakers were not well-equipped with the maturity and resources to deal with big emotions themselves. Therefore, I inherited their dysfunctional coping mechanisms.

So, what did I do? I always talk about how our children do what we do, not what we say. Unbeknown to my conscious mind, I had subconsciously inherited – I still struggle with this today – the need to dissociate when things get too hard for me. Instead of confronting myself, allowing myself to feel the pain, and, thus, helping myself heal, I dissociate. Now it occurs less often, and I know when it is happening, but I would be lying to you and, more importantly, to myself if I said it never happens.

So many of my mothering errors are inherent. They are things I have subconsciously learned through watching my tribe, the people in my close vicinity, and how they dealt with their shortcomings and calami-ties. It takes a lot of courage, resilience, authenticity, and vulnerability to heal generational trauma. But what else is the goal of existence if it is not to break through all the walls that keep us away from connecting to the spiritual realm, to the Creator, in the most sincere and authentic way possible?

Al-Ghazali has a beautiful book called *Al-Ghazali on Disciplining the Soul and on Breaking the Two Desires: Books XXII and XXIII of the Revival of the Religious Sciences.* He implies that obsessive food consumption is as much of an addiction and as detrimental to the body as sex addiction.[48] Many 'religious' people – or those of us who hold religion close to our hearts and practise and preach internally or outwardly – are very critical of addictions such as sex, drugs, and alcohol. We know, as Ghazali explains, that all addictions are but one. People just express them differently. Gabor Maté beautifully elaborates on this in his book, *Scattered Minds: The Origins and Healing of Attention Deficit Disorder*, where he speaks of trauma being the key concept that creates the dissociation.[49]

I am addicted to dissociating when things get tough. You may be addicted to numbing your sorrows with the next cheesecake or packet of chips. Others may drink intoxicants, smoke, or use pain relief pharmaceuticals or anti-stress drugs. Many of us are addicted to social media. We take our phones to the toilet because God forbid that for one split second we have the opportunity to connect with our authentic selves and, thus, connect with our hurt. All of us are trying to band-aid the same pain; we are just using different vehicles to do it. You may use sex, while I use disconnection. She uses food, and he uses street drugs. We are judgemental of the other because, in essence, we are judgemental of ourselves, which is why what presents as criticism is merely a reflection of unhealed parts within us. The pain is the same; the trauma is the same; the inability to connect with the pain is the same, but the vehicle is different. Therefore, the vehicle disadvantages the spiritual and physical bodies in different ways, but, in essence, it is merely a different catalyst used for the same equation.

Self-Worth and Addiction

My self-worth does not always come from me. I do not look in the mirror and say, "Julide, you're so beautiful. You're so smart. You're so clever." As a matter of fact, up until a handful of years ago, my self-worth came from everything and everyone but me. Previously, if someone criticised me, told me I was not a good practitioner, or said that I was a bad mum, I believed them. I would spend endless hours playing the same message in my mind, crying, finding ways to dissociate because the pain was too unbearable.

My sense of worth was attached to what others thought of me. This is why we get so worked up when someone swears at us or insults us – because we believe them. We deeply agree with them because it is what we have been brought up with: conditional love, to be worthless unless we earn our worth through academic achievements, charity work, or some other worthy endeavour. No one gave us a medal for resting and recuperating, for using time to self-discover and heal.

A lack of self-worth is the perfect breeding ground for addiction.

Many of us are addicted to praise, which means we often only do things if others can validate them. For example, we might brag about giving excessive amounts of money to charity, share how well we feed our children on social media, and tell the world that we only eat organic. This all stems from an unhealthy adult model. Of course, giving to charity and feeding ourselves and our families good food is *good*. However, the fact that these actions only occurred due to our need for praise makes them disingenuous and harmful to our sense of self-worth if it stems from there, and most of the time it does.

Think about a time you did something 'good'. If no one was looking, would you still complete this good deed? If you answered yes, would you feel better about yourself if someone praised you for doing it?

We should not need to share every piece of our lives, but we do because our insecurities stem from the fact that we do not have love for ourselves, so we need the love of others to drive us. This is partly why we are so addicted to social media. We get a sense of self-righteous satiation from other people clapping us on because we have not been taught how to love ourselves otherwise.

In the case of social media, a lot of us overshare without awareness. We think we do it because we are helping others and leading by example. We think we are growing a community of people who are inspired by the way we raise our children, the food we eat, the lifestyle we choose. But let's be real – the reason we do it is so we can receive recognition through someone else or to satiate our own sense of self-worth. When we have low self-worth, other, more dangerous addictions can start to creep in.

Why do we have cycles of binge eating? Because we go to food for the biochemical hit. Yes, food activates biochemical pathways in our brains that help to make hormones that temporarily aid us in feeling good, and we need to feel good because it is the only way to survive. So, we use food, drugs, or alcohol to help us get that hit.

Imagine that you had an argument with your partner. You both started yelling and screaming, neither of you willing to empathise with the other. The fight ended, and you buried your sorrows in Netflix and chocolate because your brain needed serotonin, the happy hormone. We cannot even sleep without it, and the only way to a quick fix biochemically is through food.

So, just like me, you dissociate from the feelings of worthlessness, helplessness, anxiety, and whatever else the argument may have left you feeling, except that you do it through food. Then when you have eaten to the point of consciously needing to vomit or not physically being able to tolerate anything else, you look at yourself in self-pity. You shame yourself. You see yourself as a worthless piece of flesh. Certain thoughts run through your mind: *Look at how weak I am. Look at me, turning to food each time. Look at me, always giving in to my addiction again and again and again.* You continue to use, so the self-perpetuating cycle of shame and self-loathing continues, slowly poisoning your spiritual and physical body each day as you take out your phone and snap a photo of your new fad diet to share on your socials.

Healing Addiction

Healing addiction is complex. I am not going to pretend that I am fully qualified to explore the ins and outs of every addiction and how it can be defeated. However, I can state a few universal truths when it comes to breaking dependence.

In my opinion, the most profound step towards healing every avenue of addiction is awareness. First, we need to know that we have a problem – "I'm addicted to drugs." "I'm addicted to food." "I'm addicted to social media." "I'm addicted to drama, sex, and alcohol." "I'm addicted to finding any way I can to disconnect from these feelings that I don't know how to deal with."

A lot of us have addictions that we are not even aware of. This is one of the reasons why we cannot make a change. Some of us are so delusional that we think we go to that charity meeting every week because we care about others – but we do not. We only care about filling a love void through helping others, and we do not even understand that this is the case. We are in complete denial and continue to assume that we act for the greater good when, in fact, we are merely satisfying the ego.

You may ask me, "Julide, are you saying we can never truly be happy about helping another or giving to the community? Is all of this just a facade, a way to satiate the ego?" No, of course it is not. Many of us do what we do because we are serving our creator through conscious living.

We genuinely want to help others. What I am saying is that in order to feel this level of authenticity and genuinely be happy for another, so many walls of pain, ego, shadows, and demons must first be conquered. How can we love another when we cannot even truly love ourselves?

And some of us just do unto others what was never done unto us. We were emotionally and physically neglected as children, so we go out and satiate everyone else's needs. Internally, we crave to have our own basic needs met. Perhaps this is why, in Islam, we understand that an intention to commit a good deed is as powerful as actually doing the deed. Because God is the owner of our manual, and, as we have inherent trauma, He is very aware that some things are not so easily actioned as they are *intended* to be actioned. In his infinite mercy, He decreed that we are rewarded equally the same.

The next step is to seek help and find the right guidance to *suit your needs.* You will need to delve into the root of what is causing your addiction before you can crush it. Never underestimate the power of support. There are many self-help books, some of which I will mention in this chapter, that will not only bring awareness to the areas in your journey that need healing, but also provide techniques and strategies to help you heal. After all, knowledge without action is futile.

One book, recommended by my business coach, that completely changed my life was *Recovery of Your Inner Child* by Lucia Capacchione. She is an arts therapist who utilises novel methods, such as using your non-dominant hand to allow your inner child to express itself. There are so many great books that hurt but heal at the same time, and this is what Allah means when he says, "Verily, with the calamity, there is ease," inna meal usri Yusra. He did not say *after* the calamity; he said *with* it. The healing is also in acknowledging that you set yourself on this journey of cleaning out the weeds in your backyard. You make your intention and hold to the ropes of Allah, and he is the one who will turn the hearts, who will bless you with the healing and watch miracles unfold.

Resources for Positive Change

There are many social media channels that share tips. As long as we know that, as conscious Muslims, what is taught is in alignment with our religious identity, we take on what fits and leave what does not. Many great self-help books exist, including *Recovery from Emotionally Immature Parents* by Lindsay C. Gibson, *The Body Keeps the Score* by Bessel van der Kolk, and *What Happened to You?* by Bruce D. Perry and Oprah Winfrey. Within each one, there is further reference to other self-help books. As long as you are aware and prepared to make active positive changes in your life, when the student is ready, the teacher will appear.

For me, this happened over ten years ago. I had hired a stand at a women's expo and had two women approach me. Back then, I did not have any awareness of my trauma, why I behaved in a particular way, or how I was triggered and why. I also had little knowledge about the personal development industry or spiritual growth and how I could approach these things in a way that aligned with my religious philosophy.

I formed a friendship with one of the women and one day while we were sipping on our lattes on Lygon Street, she asked me if I would be interested in a coach for my naturopath business. I didn't even know what a business coach was. "What do I need that for?" I asked. She offered the example of a navigation device that leads you to a particular address by telling you when and where to turn. I ended up saying yes, only because I had no boundaries and did not know how to say no. Little did I know, she would become one of the most important figures in my self-development journey and someone I would pray for in every prayer and be forever grateful for. After all, those who cannot show gratitude to another cannot show gratitude to God. In the same way, if you do not truly love yourself, you cannot truly love another.

Choosing Miracles Over Fairytales

We grow up believing in fairytales and not miracles. We grew up with Cinderella, who was an absolutely unrealistic figure. Everyone hates on her, and she forfeits her self-autonomy and sings her way through her cleaning, completely in denial and disconnected from any form of empowerment. Then there is Snow White, who is hated by her stepmother because she is more physically attractive than her. She is later kissed by a man she never consented to. Jesus, no wonder we have no bodily autonomy or boundaries. Look at all the subconscious rubbish we were subjected to as children, growing up with very neuroplastic brains. Other fairytales, such as *Little Red Riding Hood*, completely blur our perceptions of good and evil. All these stories are far from the truth, and hearing and watching them at a very young age does nothing but blur our perceptions of right and wrong, our expectations of others, our bodily autonomy, and how to hold boundaries for ourselves, to mention just a few issues. Now is the time to teach our children all of this and more, to break the cycle of generational trauma and do it as holistically, spiritually, and physically aligned as possible.

The other day, we were at a cafe, and my daughter observed her father putting some loose change into a charity box. She had a $2 coin on her and went and repeated the same behaviour as I observed her. She then came back to our table, put her head down, and started praying. "Allahim (meaning my God), please give me something too because I gave my only money to the poor people, and I really want more money under my pillow and also a rainbow cake. I hope you give these things to me." My husband and I do not oblige our children to share. We encourage, but we do not force because we want them to do everything with the proper intention and action and because they comprehend and want to, not because we forced them. My daughter looked up at me and said, "Mum, do you think Allah will give me more, because you always say we don't have to give and if we do Allah will give us more?"

To which, I replied, "One hundred percent. Allah will always give more – that's his promise in his special book. We just don't know when he will give. Maybe tomorrow, maybe ten years later, maybe when we are in heaven."

To which, she exclaimed, "In heaven! Oh my, that's a long time away, Mum!"

I responded, "Yes, it is a long time away, but we are not in charge of time. He is."

The next day she came running into the room, holding up a $20 note and saying, "Look what I found under my pillow." She asked me, "Did you put this there or did Allah?"

I said to her, "Even if I had put it there, if Allah didn't allow me, I couldn't have done it. I like to think that angels gifted that to you for your generosity."

She left the room with a massive smile on her face. As a parent, I wanted to bring awareness to the reality of miracles, not fairytales, so that on days when she feels there is no way out, no light at the end of the tunnel, she remembers that with every calamity, there is ease, and God will always make a way out for her.

CHAPTER FOUR

TRAUMA

When we hear the word 'trauma', scenes of violence, sexual abuse, and horrific accidents usually flood our minds. We think of car crashes, scenes of war, and death. Of course, these events are all traumatic. However, the trauma we are going to talk about in this book is different. The trauma I speak of is perhaps something we inflict on our children and even one another every single day without being aware that we are in fact doing it.

Trauma, as Gabor Maté puts it, is **"the invisible force that shapes our lives.** It shapes the way we live, the way we love and the way we make sense of the world. It is the root of our deepest wounds."[50]

To have trauma does not necessarily mean that we spend every day crying, agonising over the past, though some of us may do this from time to time. Experiencing the residual effects of trauma can be as simple as becoming triggered and reacting to something or someone in a specific way or demonstrating behaviour that is shaped by an event – or events – in our past. Whether consciously or unconsciously, we all react this way around the clock.

So, let me give you some examples of the type of trauma I am referring to. You were four years old and when you were crying, you were told to "shut up" before you had processed your emotions, and you never learned what to do with these feelings aside from suppress them, hide them, and lock them away, and pretty much shut up as you were told. Or perhaps you fell and cried and instead of having a caretaker give you the space to feel the pain, you were distracted with, "Oh, look, airplane." Or your pain was dismissed as something unimportant with, "Oh, look, it's not even bleeding. It's not a big deal." Or you were shamed for your response: "Don't be a sook. It's not even a big cut." These are just a few ways that your caretaker may have handled the situation, potentially creating trauma for you around trusting yourself because you were so little when you were told you were wrong. You were hurting, but your caretaker told you it was only a small cut.

You may read these lines and say, "Wait a minute. What's wrong with that? That's what I do with my kids. I distract them because I don't want them to cry or feel pain." In fact, you do not want them to acknowledge their pain because you do not know any different. You assume that anything that is painful and uncomfortable should be ignored or dismissed because that is the right thing to do. But is it? Without awareness, you do not know that what you are doing is counterintuitive to your original intention. You do not want your child to cry because you are triggered by any crying child. Why? Because you were not taught how to handle emotions, such as sadness and grief, when you were younger. Instead, you were taught to band-aid your emotions with distraction or shame or being told how to feel. This is simply because most of our caretakers did not have the resources to parent and to caretake any other way; they simply implemented what they had learned.

Let me tell you a story. One day, a girl asks her mother why every time they celebrate Independence Day, they place the turkey in the oven without its tail intact. They actually throw away the tail. The mother says, "I do it because that's what I learnt from your gran."

So, the girl goes to her gran and asks her, "Why do you cut off the tail of the turkey when you're cooking it in the oven?"

Her gran says, "I actually don't know either. That's how your great nan taught me."

So, the girl goes to her great grandmother and asks, "Grandma, why do you cut the tail off the turkey when you cook it in the oven?"

To which, her great grandmother replies, "In our days, our ovens were very small, and a whole turkey wouldn't fit inside, so we would cut the tail off so the turkey would fit."

Like this, we have inherited behaviours from generations before, and we apply them with no conscious awareness of the 'why' but just because that is what is done and that is how things are dealt with.

I remember reading a book once, *Korkutarak Degil Sevdirerek Din Egitimi*, and the author, who is a psychologist by the name of Hatice Kubra Tongar, shared a memory that a client shared with her.[51] There were parts of the client's intimate life that she was very triggered by, such as when her husband hugged her to the point where she was unable to move. She also referenced other sexual experiences that were very triggering for her, relative to this loss of physical power. She found herself angry, resentful, and in tears every time she felt overpowered by him, even in a 'simple' situation, such as a strong hug. After a few sessions, they discovered that, as a child, the client's mother would tie her hands into her pants – literally put them in her pants and tie them over with the pants string – and force-feed her. As a result, anything that put her in a state where she was not in control of her physical body brought back the emotions of that time, of that very unprocessed trauma.

Evidently, trauma comes in many forms. Trauma is being force-fed dinner when you are full because "there are kids starving in Third World countries." Trauma is being coerced into undertaking extra-curricular activities that you have no interest in to feed your parents' egos. Trauma is learning that being 'you' is not enough to receive love. Trauma is learning to be what society, your parents, or care-takers expect of you in order to feel worthy of love, which you will only receive if you fit the mould. Trauma is knowing that you are not going to be loved if you are your authentic self. Therefore, to put on a facade is trauma; to live a lie is trauma; to believe the lie you are living is trauma. Trauma is when you are your authentic self, but you are told that it is not good enough. Trauma is your mother forcing you day in, day out to wear outfits that do not align with your own likes. All of these experiences shape the way we behave as adults and the adults we become.

Often, we are afraid to label our experiences as traumatic because we feel like they are not valid or painful enough to warrant it. We think that what happened to us "wasn't that bad," and we should reserve the space for those who "had it worse." In Islam, this is not considered an objective perspective on how we should perceive what happens to us and others. The prophetic way of life encourages us to look up to and be positively envious of people who are doing better than us, whether it be in their finances, their jobs, or their capacities as leaders in the community. We should be inspired to do and be more, to look down and remember that some people have it worse, and to show gratitude and thanks for all that we do have. It is about being able to see every part of the elephant and not being limited by the part that we are touching.

Trauma from an Islamic Perspective

Yes, sights of violence, conflict, and war are definitely traumatic and mould our brains, behaviours, and personalities as adults. Everyone experiences what God has decreed for them in this lifetime. As it states in the Qur'an in surah Al-Ankabut (meaning the spider), **"Do people think that they will be let go merely by saying: 'We believe,' and that they will not be tested?"** (29:2). How we react to the things that happen to us matters more than the incidents themselves. Again, we are responsible for the journey, not the end result.

There is a saying of the Holy Prophet Muhammad, peace and blessings be upon him, reported by Al-Nu'man ibn Bashir: **"The parable of the believers in their affection, mercy, and compassion for each other is that of a body. When any limb aches, the whole body reacts with sleeplessness and fever."**[52] We are in a day and age where possibly every single limb of every single believer is aching. As a result, we find it challenging to bring our heads out of the sand and look to help others, as our suffering is so challenging in and of itself.

Words weigh a lot, which is why Islam is very protective of the human heart. The Qur'an says that when one slanders, it is as though he has bitten the flesh of his own brother, yet few of us do not slander. Slander adds to trauma, of course. When you already feel insecure, unloved, and are only able to fill your empty cup with recognition from others, their words are powerful enough to influence your thoughts and your life. As a result, the words of others can be detrimental to your spiritual and physical wellbeing. Allah says he is the one with the hearts that are torn, and to talk poorly of another is merely a reflection of the part of you that you dislike.

Acknowledging Trauma

I invite you to take a few seconds now to acknowledge your trauma. If something has had a lasting emotional, psychological, or physical impact on you, then it is trauma and must be recognised. It is only then that the process of healing can begin. Sometimes the trauma is inherited, and other times we have the emotions stored in the conscious minds, but the subconscious stores the memory. We may not recollect the memory, but the feeling, the anxiety triggered, is certainly there.

I read a book recently called *What Happened to You?: Conversations on Trauma, Resilience, and Healing*, authored by Dr Bruce Perry, in which he is asked questions by Oprah Winfrey.[53] In this book, he speaks about a boy who was in a home because his mother had passed and his father was an abusive alcoholic. This child, for some reason, did not get along with one of his teachers. Every time he encountered the teacher, he reacted with aversion, screaming at him and attacking him for no apparent reason. Lo and behold, later on, we discover that this man was wearing the same scent as his alcoholic father, so every time his brain acknowledged that scent, the emotions of resentment, hatred, anger, and remorse came to the surface.

When we have a traumatic experience – whatever it may be – every piece of associated information is stored. For example, if your parents have a fight with someone at a cafe and there is a plate of spaghetti bolognaise, a white dress, the smell of a floral perfume, and a particular song playing in the background, you may not recall the exact memory, but the emotions are attached to the subconscious. So, whenever you see spag bol, you have an aversion to that food, or a particular song makes you sick in the stomach, or you refuse to wear a white dress from that moment on. Deep, I know. Awareness is everything, so, like Alice, let us continue to go down the rabbit hole.

When was the last time someone said something that triggered you so much? Anger is really a facade for sadness, so let us talk about the last time you felt angry because you were triggered. Gabor Maté explains this eloquently in his documentary, *The Wisdom of Trauma*.[54] I'm paraphrasing here, but he asks the host something along the lines of, "When was the last time you were angry?"

The host replies, "When I had to have some renovations done to my house and the workers didn't turn up as they said they would."

He asks the host, "How did that make you feel?"

The host replies, "Angry, like I was not important, betrayed, fooled."

He interprets the tradie's inability to keep to his word as a deliberate insult, a personal attack. Gabor continues by asking if there could be another reason why the tradie was unable to attend as he had originally promised? And so, the story goes that how we perceive what is said determines our ability to translate what is actually being conveyed.

My Own Trauma

I have carried a great deal of childhood trauma throughout my life. Much of this, I have worked through – and continue to do so – with the help of my therapist.

My parents are absolute super people. I will never *ever*, in any time frame, be able to do enough for them to make up for what they have done for me and my siblings. My parents moved heaven and earth to give their children the best lives they could. Thinking about this always makes me emotional. I feel incredibly lucky, grateful, and indebted to my parents. I am guessing I always will. Although my parents did their very best for us, this does not mean we did not face challenges, and my most profound and traumatising experience relates to my first moments on this earth.

My mum had six kids – me being the eldest – within a ten-year period. She did not want to fall pregnant and when she did, from a religious perspective, abortion was not an option. When I was a newborn, Mum was depressed due to the financial and emotional hardships she was experiencing, and her labour was extremely painful. I experienced a forceps birth, so the emotional and physical pain was overpowering and perhaps did not allow her to connect with her newborn the way she would have liked. She was only able to breastfeed me for two months. According to Mum, I cried for 40 days straight. Every night, she placed a pillow on her feet and rocked me back and forth until I stopped crying from fatigue. Of course, deep down, she held resentment for this newborn baby that gave her no rest.

When I was about to turn three, my mum, my dad, my brother – who was born just ten months after me – and I migrated from Turkey to Australia. Imagine the hardship, moving to a foreign country, leaving your loved ones behind – a country whose language has never sung in your ears, whose people you have never met before. Carrying a huge amount of fear and anxiety about the present and the future is understandable. It still brings tears to my eyes today when writing this, and it will until my spirit leaves my body, for, perhaps, it enables me to empathise with others who have had a similar birthing experience.

As a result of my mother having another child ten months after I was born and four more in a short span of time, I felt emotionally abandoned and always felt the need to do things to get my parents' attention. I remember like it was yesterday that we had two Juki machines at home, as my parents were sewing basic cotton shirts for $0.50 a piece. In an attempt to get attention from my mother, I kept purposely hitting my head on the machine. Imagine the desperation a child needs to feel to physically hurt themselves in order to get crumbs of attention.

Between me and my brother, I was the quiet one. He was the one who exposed his rage. He was labelled 'the naughty child', and I was the 'the good girl' because I always shut up. I always did what I thought I needed to do for attention, which mostly involved suppressing my own needs, keeping quiet, and staying invisible. After all, Mum had five other kids to deal with. The truth is that we both had the same basic need to be seen by our parents, to be unconditionally loved. However, we both reacted in different manners to get what we needed.

As a result, I became a people pleaser. I put everyone else's needs before my own, and I had no connection with my inner child or authentic self. I found comfort, a level of self-esteem, and happiness in only giving to others because I did not know how to give to myself. Even when I considered giving to myself, I realised at a very young age that this was a pointless pursuit, as I was unimportant. Just as most of you may have done or may be doing now, consciously or unconsciously, I worked to get high grades and a 'good' career. I did everything I thought I needed to do in order to be loved by others because I never knew how to love myself. Therefore, the way to fill that void was by doing more and being more: an endless rat-race where no matter what I did, it was never enough. *I* was never enough.

I do not seek to blame my parents or my siblings or my upbringing, for that matter, or those who were involved in shaping my childhood, but I do want to share my experience. Our past experiences create the personalities we have today, and our children naturally inherit these personalities when we are not consciously parenting, when we are living life unconsciously, not really understanding why we act in a particular way or why we react to a particular thing. We just live life on autopilot, with no real acknowledgement or awareness of why we are angry or upset at something, or why we react or interact in a certain way.

We blame our parents and our circumstances a lot because it is the easiest cop-out. To point the finger at someone else not only takes away the responsibility from you, but it also takes away the empowerment and possibility of change. Imagine that someone else is the cause of your distress. How can you ever have an opportunity to heal when you leave the power in their hands? I do not write any of this to blame anyone other than myself. I acknowledge at every step of the experience that there were always opportunities for me to learn and grow. I realised I was not the victim, nor was I the villain of my lived story. I was the one who was in control of how I reacted and how I responded to my lived experiences, regardless of what they were. The responsibility was 100 percent mine, as I had free will and the ability to make a change.

Being an immigrant from a working-class family generated an entire swath of traumas I had to overcome. The expectation was that I always had to be the best academically. Love was based on – and limited by – how successful I was, how smart I was, how compliant to parental boundaries I was, how much society accepted me, and what job I did that fit society's mould. I would get 98 percent on most of my exams, and my mum's way of acknowledging me was to ask what happened to the 2 percent. This was how she was brought up: one of eight children competing for her parents' attention, learning that love had to be earned; it was not something that came naturally. So, I grew up trying to fulfil an expectation of perfectionism. Whatever I did was never good enough for myself. I never gave myself a pat on the back for my achievements. Instead, I cracked the whip even harder.

Monkey See, Monkey Do

Many people grow up in families that have experienced severe amounts of violence and conflict – significant trauma that leaves everlasting scars. But, for most of us, we have not been subjected to objectively extreme suffering. For example, we may not have experienced abuse, domestic violence, or poverty. This does not mean that we do not have trauma, that our trauma does not exist, or that our trauma is not valid or important. You matter, and you *are* important.

In *The Body Keeps the Score*, Bessel van der Kolk speaks of how trauma is stored in bodily organs and gives scientific evidence that shows how trauma can appear as a physical, chronic illness.[55] This may be one of the reasons for the increase in autoimmune illnesses.

In her book, *Loving Yourself to Great Health*, Louis Hay makes a viable connection between autoimmune illnesses and a lack of self-love. She explains the psychological manifestations of disease that stem from mental or emotional states. For example, she states that someone who experiences slow thyroid function – although they are certainly not exempt from biochemical causes, such as low iodine – could be experiencing this on a spiritual or emotional level due to being someone who was unable to speak up and say what they really wanted to say.[56] Instead, perhaps, they kept the truth inside because they were afraid of the judgement or accountability that came with it. Another thought-provoking example given in the book is that constipation is the physical manifestation of an inability to let go of emotions, such as resentment, remorse, and sadness.

Most of us have been exposed to repeated behaviour that has, over time, caused damage to our emotional, psychological, and physical wellbeing. Sadly, unless we have conscious awareness, our trauma becomes the personality of our own children. For example, in traditionally Turkish households, the mother is usually obsessively clean, an impeccable cook, and an exceptional child bearer. She holds everything together and strives for perfection in everything she does. In her mind, to be imperfect would be to fail, and to fail would be shameful. Her sense of self-worth comes from maintaining this facade, so imagine what happens to her when she cannot. She is her own biggest self-critic.

At face value, this sort of behaviour does not *sound* all that bad, right? In fact, to some, it may sound great! A mum who goes above and beyond to run an impeccable household – what could be better? However, this type of behaviour promotes unrealistic standards in our children. When we witness our parents placing such high pressure on themselves, we unknowingly pick up these benchmarks and apply them to ourselves. We think, "Gee, Mum is so perfect. This is how a woman needs to be." But it does not show us the full story. What we see is what we do so when we see parents who are 'always together' emotionally, we do not allow ourselves to feel sad, or disappointed, or upset, or any emotion that may not have been shown to us by our caretakers.

Then, when we have our own families, we replicate our parents' behaviour. Suddenly, we are the ones who must be impeccably neat and tidy and great cooks. Then we spend our whole lives striving for perfection, which we eventually realise does not exist, while our kids watch on. Eventually, they too inherit this unrelenting desire for perfection, and the cycle continues. No one realises that the impeccable household will meet suffering via another avenue. More than likely, self-care will be neglected, or your partner and their needs will be left behind. But that is okay, because the public will only ever see your house and food.

In the Islamic culture, the woman's only job once she is a parent is to raise her children in the best way possible. As a matter of fact, in many Middle Eastern countries, such as Saudi Arabia, it is a necessity not a luxury to have a housekeeper who performs all the cooking and cleaning so the mother can nurture her children properly without the additional burdens that society puts on her. Religiously, all that is asked of a mother is to bring up righteous children. Anything done outside of this may accumulate brownie points, but it is in no way a religious obligation.

During our formative years, our parents are our biggest influence. When we have our own families, much of our parenting is unconscious, as we usually parent the same way that our parents did, unless we have conscious awareness. Why? Because that is all we saw. It is a completely natural and common occurrence, and it is not always a bad thing. Maybe your dad taught you how to be more compassionate, or your mum instilled in you a strong work ethic. These are good traits that you can pass on to your kids. However, with the good comes the not so good. If we do not put in the work and turn our minds to the unhealthy behaviours that our parents passed on to us, we will continue the cycle of trauma by passing these traits on to the next generation. It is up to us to think about the kinds of parents we want to be, which should only ever align with the utmost compassion, love, and mercy that our prophet showed his children. We each must acknowledge and heal our own traumas so we do not unconsciously inflict our unresolved pain on *our* children.

Although I was a people pleaser as a teenager, Mum also gave me other traits. She is an avid reader, and my love of reading comes from her. She also forced me out of my comfort zone with public speaking, giving me the confidence and push I needed to perform at events and become a public speaker. She gave me my religious values, which kept me safe as a child and teenager. Even when my parents were not watching, I knew that God was, and my love for him – although there was a lot of fear of

God instilled in us before love – prevented me from looking to fill a void with addictions. She taught me how to be a compassionate, empathetic sister, how to take care of my siblings, and how to be a caring mother. She taught me to ensure I was on my own feet, to have financial freedom, to be a strong community leader, to lead by example. My mother taught me much of the strength and perseverance I have today. She taught me I can get to the top, just like anyone else. My mother taught me that a woman is stronger than society makes her believe she is. My mother kept nudging me out of my comfort zone to help me build the resilience and strength I have today as a community leader.

I do not deny that I felt a massive emotional void as a child. I felt emotionally neglected because just like many parents, mine were in survival mode. They put a roof over our heads and gave us hot food and safety, but they were emotionally neglected too by parents who were also emotionally neglected. Do you see the cycle? Where there is no awareness, there is no room for change. A survival mindset inherited from our ancestors, who experienced World War I and II, made my parents believe that these things were all that were necessary to bring up a child and that the emotional side was not important. Even if it were, how do you raise six children with emotional fullness? Perhaps understanding my mother is not about justifying the emotional shortcomings I experienced as a child, but in understanding the reasons behind her actions. Instead of being laser-focused on the things that became the foundation of the dysfunctional personality within me, I could make space in my heart to acknowledge, forgive, and adopt a more objective view of my childhood experiences. Perhaps that is the best way forward. Islamically, this is where divine destiny draws the line. This is where I look back at my childhood and know that it was exactly the childhood I had to live to become the woman I am today.

Consequences of Childhood Neglect

Due to the emotional neglect I experienced as a child, I unconsciously wanted to give my daughter what I did not have myself: unconditional love, care, compassion, and time – which actually caused anxiety for her. As a first-time parent, I spent every minute with her because I thought no one else was good enough and no one else would do for her what I could do. I did this at the cost of my own physical and mental health, and my social life.

One day, when Elisa was one and a half years old, I realised how much separation anxiety she had and acknowledged that the stepping stone to this anxiety was actually *my* separation anxiety, my unrelenting standards, and the perfectionistic attitude I had. After all, I was not worthy of love or being titled a good mum unless I was perfect, right? To me, perfect meant doing everything for her without reaching for help, at the cost of burnout. It is very important to look at ourselves and how we are raising our children, considering our own upbringing and in which areas we need to heal. I thought that giving her everything meant burning the candle at both ends. I was so scared of creating the emotional void in her that I had as a child that I had no boundaries at all. I was overly protective of her, hardly allowing her any opportunities to develop resilience and create boundaries. Once I acknowledged how incorrect I was in my approach, I made very serious changes.

Mind you, Mum and I talk about emotional neglect all the time. Mum says that she learnt from her own mother to care from a perspective of fear. If she instilled enough fear in us, she could control us, meaning that nothing would happen to us, which was her biggest fear as a woman raising six children in a country so foreign to her. It makes so much sense. She wanted to ensure that her kids were safe at the cost of anything, and this was the only way she knew how to parent until she actively started practicing Islam. Then she changed.

Practicing Islam consciously in a non-Muslim country gave her the perspective she needed and removed the unnecessary and traumatising cultural parenting that she was inflicting on her children. I will forever be grateful to a woman who, regardless of her upbringing, once she realised the errors in her parenting, was not arrogant or egocentric. She knew that change was necessary, so she embarked on that painful journey of realising her own mistakes and healing from her own traumas.

In contrast to Elisa, my son, Alparslan, is so independent, has the most vibrant personality, and his level of resilience and self-confidence shines through. He slept in his own bed a lot sooner than his sister, and he was happy to see me when I got home but not anxious when I left him. I learned and healed from the co-dependent relationship I'd had with my daughter, and these problems did not reflect in my son.

Now, do I blame myself? No, I do not. Instead, I acknowledge that I laid the foundations of her anxiety by parenting the way I did. The minute I had awareness, and as much as I knew healing would be painful, I went in headfirst. I acknowledged that I would never purposely create any trauma in my children – as no parent or caretaker would ever purposely do – and did my best to accept my own shortcomings and work on them. As a result, I now have an independent young daughter, whose boundaries are a lot better than mine and can say to her Montessori tutor, who offered her hand sanitiser, "No thanks, we don't use chemicals on our hands. I will go wash my hands."

And when her Montessori tutor told her brother to "stop crying," she stood up to her 50-odd-year-old tutor in confidence and was able to say, "Actually, Margaret, Mum taught us to feel all of our emotions, so we don't say stop crying to each other. We can just hug each other, wait till the person feels better, and allow them to feel safe so they can stop crying when they are ready."

She also has the confidence to hold a religious boundary and tell her tutor that we are Muslim and we do not eat pork. And, most recently, at our local play centre, a child repeatedly threw balls at her even though she asked him to stop. How did my daughter react? She came to me and said she would be having a word with the child's parents. Then she approached the parent and asked them to help their child understand not to hit her with balls. "I did ask him a few times, and he didn't respond to me, so I wanted to tell you" she explained.

So many of us grow up with no bodily autonomy in our culture. "Kiss your uncle's hand."

"Don't be rude, hug your aunty."

"Say thank you, you're being very unkind!" as though a forced thank you makes a difference when the child is not able to actually mean what they say.

In my clinic, every single woman I have ever worked with who has had a reproductive issue has had a history of boundary invasion – they have either been sexually or physically molested. All this comes from our pervasive culture, which forces children to kiss hands, sit on the laps of uncles, and hug 'relatives'. Elisa and Alp do not like to hug hello or kiss goodbye. I have taught them body autonomy, and they are able to say, "I don't want a hug." Instead, they say, "But if you want, I can high five you." This is incredibly important because I know as I write these lines, many of you will be in tears because you have had someone who is related to you touch you inappropriately. It is your secret to the grave because you hold on to the shame as though it is your fault – but it is not. It is due to the unfortunate lack of resources your parents had, which led to you not learning body autonomy or creating boundaries. Instead, you were at the mercy of any souls who had a *nafs*, an ego.

Sometimes, my inner people pleaser kicks in as I watch Elisa tell her grandad that she won't be hugging him today, or when she doesn't want to thank someone for a gift they have purchased for her, or when she sets boundaries and says she doesn't want to go on a play date with a friend who is asking, or when I watch her tell someone that she doesn't want to play with them. Oh man, my inner people pleaser burns and says, *Just do it, Elisa, make them feel happy too*, as though my Elisa is responsible for their emotions. She isn't, but we grow up feeling emotionally responsible for how others feel. I thank God that my inner voice isn't heard because my healed adult tells my inner child that Elisa has a right to respectfully hold boundaries. She has a right over her body and even though this is displeasing for the most part, and perhaps in our culture she is even viewed as a disrespectful child, I secretly am so proud of her resilience.

My job is not finished, but I am so proud of how far I have come as a mother, and I acknowledge that every part of me that continues to heal reflects in my children. To God, I am forever grateful for the opportunity to turn inwards and do the work that I would otherwise have been oblivious too, the work that inspired me to write this book. By sharing my own experiences, traumas, and vulnerabilities, perhaps you will find some level of inspiration and actively make changes in your own life.

Conscious Parenting

To be a conscious parent is to look inward at our own baggage and triggers and ensure that they are healed to the best of our abilities.

Conscious parents respect their children and treat them as individuals, not as extensions of themselves. When I was young, I knew that the only way to receive love was to be what my mum wanted me to be. I tried to be exactly that, even though it conflicted with my own authentic self, until one day I woke up drowning in my own tears and sorrows. Eventually, I acknowledged that change had to come – I could not keep up this facade.

As conscious parents, conscious Muslims, and conscious humans, as the vicegerents the Qur'an likes to refer to us as, rather than making our children conform to a predetermined list of standards, we give them the space to grow and lean into their authentic selves. The child-parent relationship is viewed as a two-way street, as opposed to the disciplinarian-submissive binary that is more common in traditional parenting styles, which most of us are familiar with.

Everyone has their own style of parenting, and that is okay. But what you need to think about is *why* you are rearing your kids in a certain way. For example, why are you sending your child to timeout as punishment? Is that really the best way to teach them right from wrong? Or is it because you cannot handle the fact that your child said no to you, so you oppress them because that is what you saw when you said no to your parents? The quickest way to deal with an opposing view is to censor it, oppress it, take away the voice. But what if you allowed it to have a voice to better understand it? What if you asked "why?" and got curious as to why your child said no to you? Did they say no to bedtime because you spent the whole day drowning your own sorrows by disassociating yourself in cleaning; therefore, they have so much physical energy left that they were not able to expend? Or perhaps they do not find their mattress comfortable or are scared in their bedroom. How are you to ever know the reason for the 'no' unless you ask?

In my teenage life, I resented religion so much. I was 16 and attended a particular mosque where the teacher never allowed me or my cousin to read the Qur'an because we were slow readers, so she just chose the girls who were better at reciting. At this age, my people-pleasing times were over – it was time to rebel. All that suppressed emotion was coming to the surface with a vengeance. I complained every day in the car about how much I hated going to Islamic school on Sundays, but it made no difference to Mum because she knew I would still do what I was told to do. Once I found my own path back home, I learned to love religion and realised that the resentment I had felt was not towards the religion itself but for the cultural misogyny that paraded as religion – but it was far from it.

Reflecting on it now, I acknowledge that the teacher loved to make those girls read because, in a way, they made her feel better about herself. She did not call on me because I could not read properly. But, to her, the ones who could were the result of her work and, thus, fed her ego. Perhaps that was how she filled her self-worth void.

I had to spiritually leave religion to find my path again, to understand that what was portrayed as religion was a poor attempt at cultural oppression, and that God's mercy was mentioned hundreds of times over his wrath in the Qur'an. However, the schools spoke about his wrath first. What better way to control a population of people than to create fear in them? After all, fear is a huge driver of the human collective, something that absolutely takes away conscious and critically constructive thinking. I had a scarf on my head but a massive spiritual void in my heart. No one knew about it because, superficially, everyone saw a girl in a scarf, and a scarf meant religious identity.

I speak of conscious parenting as a loose term to encompass our religious and moral expectations from the Islamic tradition. A religion whose prophet would stand up and give his seat to his own daughter, a religion whose prophet never laid a finger on his children, a religion whose prophet never yelled or raised his voice and always came from a place of empathy, a religion whose prophet responded to a man who told him he never hugged his children with, "What can I do if God has made your heart void of love?"

Being fond of children, Prophet Muhammad showed great interest in playing with them. His involvement in children's games shows us the great importance in playing with our children.

He would have fun with the children who came back from Abyssinia and tried to speak with them in Abyssinian. It was his practice to give lifts on his camel to children when he returned from journeys. Prophet Muhammad never held back his love for the children and always expressed his fondness to them. In one Hadith, Abu Hurairah (may Allah be pleased with him) narrated:

> I went along with Allah's Messenger (peace and blessings be upon him) at a time during the day but he did not talk to me and I did not talk to him until he reached the market of Banu Qaynuqa.
>
> He came back to the tent of Fatimah and said, **"Is the little chap (meaning Al-Hasan) there?"** We were under the impression that his mother had detained him in order to bathe and dress him and garland him with sweet garland.
>
> Not much time had passed that he (Al-Hasan) came running until both of them embraced each other, thereupon Allah's Messenger (peace and blessings be upon him) said, **"O Allah, I love him; love him and love one who loves him."** (Muslim)
>
> Anas ibn Malik (may Allah be pleased with him), the servant of the Prophet, had another recollection: **I never saw anyone who was more compassionate towards children than Allah's Messenger (peace and blessings**

be upon him). His son Ibrahim was in the care of a wet nurse in the hills around Madinah. He would go there, and we would go with him, and he would enter the house, pick up his son and kiss him, then come back. (Muslim)[57]

If this was the example set by the epitome of mankind, whose footsteps are we really following when we hit our children, yell at them, and punish them? For the most part, each one of us is an unloved child stuck in an adult's body – a child who has only ever been hurt, thus, only ever learned to hurt back. This was not really mirrored to us growing up. As mentioned earlier, I remember that our weekend Islamic school teacher would usually skip me when we were reciting the Arabic script because I never studied it, and I read it very slowly. She never bothered creating a way to help me love Islam or to make it more enjoyable for me and instead would instil fear in our hearts about what we should not do and what the punishment would be. The wrath of God was embedded in our hearts before His love for us, even though his mercy is mentioned close to 400 times in the book as opposed to his wrath being mentioned fewer than 100.

Interestingly, in Islam, formal education does not commence for the child until they are 7–8 years old, which coincides with the development of the prefrontal cortex. It is not even appropriate to teach a child of God's wrath or the existence of hell before the age of seven because they do not have the ability to fully comprehend. Thus, the information given will only be fear-based, and fear only lasts so long.

The Language of Crying

There is a whole school of thought around controlled crying. Essentially, controlled crying involves letting your child cry it out and settle themselves rather than comforting them immediately when they are unsettled and trying to sleep.

Some parents opt for this method to help get a baby into a sleep routine quickly. However, this goes against any form of common sense, as a baby does not know how to comfort or soothe itself. That part of the prefrontal cortex is not yet developed, yet the baby eventually submits out of the fatigue from crying or out of desperation because no one is responding to the only way it knows how to get attention.

Studies confirm that controlled crying methods put babies' and toddlers' cortisol levels through the roof, which can actually contribute to an inability to control temper and an inability to be more calm and grounded due to the overuse of the sympathetic nervous system.[58]

We are taught that kids are wily. Do not sleep with your child, he is playing with you. Do not respond kindly when he cries, he is just trying to manipulate you. Do not pick him up, he will get used to being in your lap. However, the people who say these things have no understanding of neuroscience and, of course, likely did not have a parent who held space for them. Therefore, not only do they not hold space for their own children, but they also have no awareness around how destructive this behaviour is.

Now, it is not up to me to tell you how to parent your babies, but it is important to be mindful and introspective in whatever methods or approaches you use. In *Scattered Minds*, Gabor Maté sheds light on this matter, sharing literature that confirms that the trauma brain forms in utero and in the first 18 months of our lives.[59] When we cry and we are ignored, we are ignored in the only language we know how to speak. We are taught quickly that if we raise a concern and it does not align with our parents' priorities, we will not be heard, and we will not be responded to. We are alone.

If ignoring a baby's cries increases cortisol levels and, therefore, stress, it is no wonder that our children are diagnosed with ADD or ADHD and are so angry, and why they do not know how to safely express their emotions. In fact, there has been a physical biochemical shift in the way their brains have developed, due to our neglect.

One study shows that controlled crying can reduce pre-sleep behavioural cues of distress – that is, crying – in infants by the third day of practice. However, cortisol levels remain the same, indicating that the feelings of distress are still present, but the children are no longer vocalising their concerns.[60] I am sure any parents who understood this would also be feeling distress knowing that their children were not calling out when they were suffering and in need. In a position statement that references the study mentioned, the Australian Association for Infant Mental Health (AAIMH) advises that infants and young children waking throughout the night and needing attention is "normal" and "healthy." The report states that responding to a child's cries does not create bad habits but does, in fact, improve their sense of security.[61]

Self-Love and Healthy Boundaries

As discussed, your children will copy you. The science is called mirror neurons. Let me explain this, as it does not just relate to children. We have mirror neurons that affect us and how we behave as adults, depending on who we are around. Scientifically speaking, "Mirror neurons are a class of neuron that modulate their activity both when an individual executes a specific motor act and when they observe the same or similar act performed by another individual."[62] In lay terms, we copy the behaviours we are most subjected to. So, when you show your children that life is only about sacrificing yourself and compromising your personality and your physical and emotional needs for others, you are teaching them to act this way. Perhaps this is the key reason why we become people pleasers and why we put the needs of others above our own. We see our parents exhibit this behaviour; we then unconsciously depict and reflect the same behaviour in our own lives. Acknowledging this is the first step toward healing.

The second step is making a change. It is like when Islam asks you to tailor every other need around your five daily prayers. For example, you do not pray when you have time; you make time during the day to fulfil your five obligatory prayers around your other commitments. In Islam, this is self-love. Putting aside time to wash your body, pray to align yourself, and clear your mind is, in essence, what the West sees as self-love or self-care. It is more than this; however, Islamically, this is literally the least we need to do.

Some people will take this to mean that we are to put ourselves before others, but Islam teaches us selflessness and putting others first. Islam endorses keeping our luxuries to a minimum and eating not until we are full, but one third of our stomach. Islam enforces the importance of maintaining our physical and mental health by telling us what and when to consume. Prophet Muhammad (PBUH) teaches us through his life what it means to preserve our energy, use our energy for good, for ourselves, and for others. He also teaches us what rest is.

The Prophet Muhammad once asked a companion: "(Is it true) that you fast all day and stand in prayer all night?" The companion replied that the report was true. The Prophet then said: "Do not do that! Observe the fast sometimes and also leave (it) at other times. Stand up for prayer at night and also sleep at night. Your body has a right over you, your eyes have a right over you and your wife has a right over you."[63]

In the previous chapter, we briefly talked about the concept of self-worth. Let us tease this out a little. When we have low self-worth and self-love, we are unable to regulate our emotions when we are challenged, when we make a mistake, or when we fail. These events often send us 'over the edge' as thoughts like *I'm hopeless*, *I'm worthless*, *I'm such a screw-up* cloud our minds. We blame and chastise ourselves, finding it impossible to self-forgive. When we live to please others, we are unable to cope as soon as someone is unhappy with or critical of us. The moment we base our value on how others treat us, we hand over control of our happiness. This can cause all sorts of problems. Let me share a story.

A Welcome Epiphany about Self-Worth

Once, I had an epiphany that related to a confrontation I had with a client. It blew my socks off, and, in hindsight, I *thank God* that it happened. The conflict gave me the opportunity to acknowledge my own lack of self-worth and make many changes within myself. The client experienced chronic migraines, so we performed a hair sample, which showed that she had very high levels of mercury in her system. This led me to the scientific assumption that mercury could be the cause of the problem.

We started a mercury detox, and her migraines became less frequent. Eventually, they disappeared entirely, replaced by slight headaches when she ate too much sugar or was dehydrated, which are common headache causes. Alongside this, the client was suffering from multiple infections: one in her colon, one in her stomach, and one in her small intestine. I recommended that she eat less sugar to combat the infections, or else they would persist. I also gave her some other dietary and lifestyle advice and supplements to take. As with many clients, the dietary changes were the hardest to implement, especially reducing her sugar intake.

I explained to her that bacteria thrive on sugar; they use glucose to multiply; thus, it would be counterintuitive to continue eating a diet full of refined sugars while taking botanical antimicrobials at the same time. She was also very stressed, and cortisol does not help when you are warding off infection, as it suppresses the immune system. The body thinks it is in danger, and warding off this danger is more important than repairing the body. The more ramped-up your stress hormones are, the less likely you are to heal from an infection, as cortisol is an immune-suppressing hormone.[64]

One day, during a consultation, my client started crying and told me that I was the reason why she was not pregnant. She believed that I had delayed her ability to recover. It was all my fault because I was not doing enough to change her health.

Now, the first thing I should have done was ground myself in my own knowledge, the knowledge that the body will only go at the pace that it is able. No practitioner can speed that up. The only person who can speed up the process is *the client*, depending on how consistently they follow the recommended strategies. The practitioner may navigate but if the practitioner asks the client to turn right and they turn left, they are not going to get the desired results. I should have stood my ground and reconfirmed that the very thing she had admitted to – ice cream or something sweet every other night, high stress levels due to recently losing a loved one, and issues with her husband – were all creating detours as she worked towards her ultimate goal. But I did not stand my ground. Instead, I cried.

My sense of self-worth came from how successful I was in my clinic, and, 99 percent of the time, I was very successful. However, when I got the odd client who vomited negativity on me because they were not improving, I felt unable to cope – like I was a failure, a disappointment, not good enough.

She's right, I thought. Why *can't I make her better?* All this time, all this money, all this energy – it was all my fault. Why could I not have thought of a better plan, found another company or other products, invented another solution? It was not her fault. I should have known better. I should have *done* better. My traumatised child belief system re-emerged: not being good enough, not being deserving of love, and everything being my fault.

In this woman's case, her refusal to see a psychologist ultimately impeded her progress. She had trauma around food. I advised her that the only way forward was to see a therapist – the way she behaved around food would only change if she acknowledged *why* she had an emotional connection to it in the first place. But she would not do it. She refused, saying that she was not willing to see a therapist as she thought it would not make a difference. She would not accept that the responsibility was on her to stop consuming sugar, which could only happen after she dealt with her food trauma with the help of a qualified psychologist. As a practitioner, I could have said, "This is what needs to be done and if you are not currently aligned with my treatment plan, then perhaps you need to see an alternative practitioner who may be on the same wavelength." But I did not do that.

Every statement she made to me, I took completely to heart. My negative inner voice took over. *You're not good enough. You couldn't get this patient well*, my unrelenting standards barked at me. *It has been one and a half years, and you're still not where you should be. Why hasn't this client gotten pregnant, Julide? She said you were too expensive, and she's right. You're not worth it.* I felt inadequate because my client had not achieved the results she wanted.

The first thing I needed to acknowledge with my therapist was that I was not responsible for *anyone's* level of health success, good or bad. As much as it was not my fault if people did not achieve their desired results, it was also not to my victory if they did. If I say turn right and the client does, then all credit goes to them. Supplements do not magically take themselves, and lifestyle changes do not miraculously happen. It is the investment of time, money, and knowledge that really gets results. I accepted that I am not the creator of all my patients' good outcomes. The real heroes are the ones who take on the advice, apply the changes, persevere, and watch the miracles in their mental and physical health unfold.

On the flip side, if clients are not getting good results, I am also not to blame. It is not on me if they do not make the necessary changes. Outcomes do not just happen. You cannot simply pop a pill for a couple of months and expect to get results. Your sense of self-worth should only come from within. If it comes from an external factor, it is always going to be up and down. This can be very fatiguing on the nervous system. It was not until I acknowledged that my own sense of self-worth was attached to others, and healed this part of me, that I was truly able to love and value myself. It was only then that I truly became liberated from my chains of conditioning, because my sense of confidence, self-worth, and self-esteem came from within. Who we are in our authentic selves matters most, and it is important for this to be aligned with our spiritual stance – all else is background noise.

Islam and Increasing Self-Worth

How do we increase self-worth if we do not see a psychologist and work on the very childhood wounds that created that inner voice, that void we are only able to fill with the confirmation and acknowledgement of others?

When we look at it from an Islamic perspective, we are followers of a religion whose first verse revealed was "read" and whose last message was "we have completed this religion for you." To me, that meant I had to be curious and courageous enough to unlearn when necessary. It meant showing humility when learning, admitting what I did not know, and having the integrity and humbleness to admit to being wrong in a society where being wrong was frowned upon.

So, how do we build self-respect and self-love within the paradigm of Islam? Firstly, we must acknowledge and understand where our trauma is coming from. Perhaps the low self-esteem stems from childhood. Perhaps your parents or someone else bullied you and put you down. Perhaps, as an adult, you experienced poor performance in a job, or a failed marriage or relationship. As a matter of fact, much of our identity comes from what others have said about us, not from what we have told ourselves. Your life circumstances are not you, and they are certainly not immutable. They can change. They are events that have happened to you with the permission of the divine; however, they do not define you. You are given the test and need to sit it. If you do not pass, then you will be presented the same test again, perhaps in a different way, but it will be presented to you.

As Allah says in the Qur'an, "Do people think once they say, 'We believe,' that they will be left without being put to the test? We certainly tested those before them. And in this way Allah will clearly distinguish between those who are truthful and those who are liars" (29:2). We acknowledge that whatever happens to us, whether we translate it as being good or bad, happens because Allah allows it to happen, and how we respond matters most.

We may think that Islam has no place for self-love because self-love is too superficial, but that is incorrect. How we live is how we model life to our little ones, and The Prophet Muhammad (PBUH) said, "None of you truly believes until he loves for his brother what he loves for himself."[65] This Hadith assumes that we love ourselves. But do we really?

Islam teaches us to show kindness, patience, compassion, and forgiveness to other people (Qur'an 4:36, 90:17, and 2:109). Do you not think we should show the same to ourselves? Our approach has always been to do more for others and neglect ourselves, and this is what has typically been taught as right, but, as in a plane in trouble, you must put on your own oxygen mask if you wish to help the next person with theirs.

God knows that man can be unjust to himself, to his own soul, and says so in the Qur'an. The Holy Qur'an describes one particular man: "And he entered his garden while he was unjust to himself" (18:35). If God states that he is able to forgive all sins, then why are we so hard on ourselves in relation to forgiving ourselves for our past lives and mistakes?

The Prophet (PBUH) said, "All the sons of Adam are sinners, but the best of sinners are those who repent often."[66]

When we are victims of our circumstances, it is disempowering. Why, you ask? Because we place the responsibility – thus, the ability for change – in the hands of others, which leaves us unable to do anything. Once we take responsibility for ourselves, our health, and our mental health wholeheartedly, we increase our level of self-respect and self-efficacy, thus, improving self-esteem. The breeding of a victim mentality causes the opposite: the loss of the ability to change and improve.

Allah says in the Qur'an: "Surely Allah does not change the conditions in which a people are in until they change that which is in themselves" (13:11). To me, this means we must first have awareness and then consciously take action. Only then will God help clear our path and help us reach our goals, whereas in the linear paradigm, for most of us, disease 'just happens'. It happens by pot luck, and that is that. We take it on the chin, with no responsibility or self-change.

One of the ways we can ensure that we are not repeating traumatic experiences for our children is to celebrate their uniqueness. We need to be comfortable with who they are, as opposed to wanting them to be who we want them to be because that is what will ultimately serve our ego. If you have ever been to an Ottoman madrasah (meaning an Islamic school), you may have seen an inscription that translates to, "Here no fish is forced to fly, and no bird asked to swim." But how do we know if our children are fish or birds if we do not spend enough time with them, if they continue to trigger us and we choose to turn away from that trigger or control and manipulate it through oppressing them or taking away their voice, if we keep their school schedules and social lives so busy they don't get a minute to turn inward and acknowledge their authentic selves?

In essence, when we look at teachings of Montessori and Steiner, they very much align with the Islamic teachings of what holistic, conscious parenting looks like, recognising that each child has their own unique gifts. Once we acknowledge what these gifts are and find ways to nurture and amplify them through intuitive play, we can effectively guide children towards their strengths. Thus, they will be more likely to align with careers that suit their personality traits.

The challenge in our schooling system is that we put the fish, the rabbit, the snail, the lion, and the elephant all in the one room and utilize one typical method of education. When we do not get the best from our children, as opposed to blaming the system that is incorrectly trying to mould them, we blame the children themselves and question their abilities. The education system refuses to create a unique model for each child and fails to meet their individual needs.

Healthy Boundaries

Our inability to set healthy boundaries with ourselves and in our relationships creates a perpetual cycle of shame and a lack of self-worth. By continually letting others encroach on our limits, we are saying to ourselves – and to them – that our value is so low that we accept being treated however they deem appropriate. This disempowers us and means we often tolerate behaviour that hurts, harms, or alienates us. What does this mean?

In my clinic, I charge the exact same fee to both clients who do and do not turn up to their consultations. This is because I value my time and respect my work, and there is no way I would get that time back. When I set time aside for a particular person, no one else can take that slot. My cancellation policy is set in stone and applied regardless of the reason for the cancellation.

Every excuse is justified: one mother might have stayed up all night with her child who has a fever; another may have had a fight with her husband; someone else might have had a very stressful week moving. Most of the time, the reasons for people missing their consultations are reasonable. However, it is not my responsibility as a practitioner to bear the consequences, regardless of how justified their reasons are. If I did that, I would compromise my own sense of self-worth and lose a whole lot of time that I could never get back. That might sound harsh, but it is my boundary. Much of the time, it *will* sound harsh to someone who does not have boundaries. To someone who does, it will seem reasonable, as, in essence, it indicates a certain level of self-respect.

As a person who now sets healthy boundaries, I am not offended when others enforce their own. I feel liberated on their behalf. It feels good to connect with people who respect themselves enough to say, "I will never get back this half an hour that has been reserved for you. I understand if you can't make it, however, there are certain consequences if you don't." Generally, the clients who happily pay the fee are the ones who have healthy boundaries. The ones who complain are usually those who do not. I cannot take responsibility for someone who may not yet have healthy boundaries in place. All I can do is live the example of my own authentic self in my own light. Some will see the light shining. For others, it will be harsh on their eyes, and they will run from it because that level of self-love and respect is too foreign to them.

When we grow up in co-dependent households that lack boundaries, we may not develop the ability to set boundaries ourselves. This is because our personalities are oppressed to the point where we are not allowed to be ourselves, and we are conditioned to not value our worth. Instead, we are groomed to behave in ways that are acceptable to others and meet cultural standards, which seem to be of more import than our religious standards.

Growing up, my mother often pushed me into things. She would say things like, "I want you to talk on that radio show because I never got the chance to" or, "I want you to read this poem because I wasn't able to." Though Mum was providing me with amazing opportunities, she was also, unknowingly, reliving her childhood trauma of not having access to those opportunities through me. I was growing up to be an extension of the unlived version of my mother rather than the authentic version of myself.

At six years old, my daughter had her own sense of style and her own dress code. It used to intimidate me because she wanted to wear things that I did not want her to be seen in public wearing. I had a certain idea about what I wanted others to think of me and my children. When I realised that I was triggered by my daughter's sense of dress, I immediately knew that I was coming from a place of ego and that I needed more healing.

Nowadays, my daughter's favourite clothing is tie-dye printed stuff, leopard print shoes, leggings, and baggy tops, and I am cool with that.

What used to bother me, I now look at with pride. I am so proud that she can shine in her own authentic light. After all, she is not an extension of me. She is her own person, and I want to continue to encourage this in alignment with my own religious and spiritual ethos.

My parents loved me unconditionally. However, as a child, I saw their love as being conditional. I always thought that they would only love me if I reached *that* goal or achieved *that* success. I did whatever I could to make them happy because I was a sucker for any crumb of love they offered. And it was not just me. We, as a human collective, are all suckers for any crumb of love or attention from our parents, loved ones, or extended communities. This is a key reason why we like to be a part of the herd as opposed to an outlier, lonely but shining our own light for ourselves. We want to feel safe, and the way to feel safe most of the time is to betray our unique, genuine, authentic selves just so we can fit society's mould.

Because I developed people-pleasing behaviours, I was unable to set boundaries. My self-worth was so attached to the happiness of others that I could not enforce my own limitations out of fear that I would disappoint someone else. My self-worth was nothing compared to the value I placed on those external to me. Also, my sense of self-worth was dependent on what other people thought about me so when people thought good things, applauded, and sung my praise, I was on cloud nine. But when the criticism came and people were not pleased with the work I was doing or my stance on a particular religious or political topic, it absolutely crushed my sense of self-worth. Growing up believing that we are only as worthy as what people think of us is what leads to this level of disaster when we reach adulthood. We expect everybody to love us, but that will never happen. And when it does not happen, it affects our mental health significantly.

With my own children, I try to acknowledge and bring out the things they like to do and their God-gifted talents. For example, my daughter loves everything to do with reading, imagination, and play, and my son loves drawing and playing ball games. My job is not to say, "I want you to do this" or, "You have to try that," but to nurture what is already within them. As a parent, it is my responsibility to discover and encourage the pearl within them that makes them unique, as opposed to servicing my own agenda or unlived dreams. As conscious parents, we should all strive to do this. This aligns with the Islamic conscious parenting agenda. As we peel back the layers of the onion in relation to the personality traits of our children, we can start to acknowledge the innate gifts they have been given by God.

We should embark on our own journeys instead of those that our parents feel are academically or financially feasible. As Muslims, the careers that our parents push us towards are not always the most prestigious or high-paying. They are the careers that our parents wanted but could not have. I understand that some parents reading this book will feel triggered, especially by this chapter. "That's not why I wanted my child to study law." "That's not why I wanted her to be a doctor." "That's not why I pushed him towards that career." But the reality is that when we continue to dig, we unearth a deeper reason behind everything we say and do. Once we acknowledge that our reasons do not always stem from a healthy place but from a void within ourselves that we wish to fill, we understand ourselves better, have much healthier relationships with our children, and absolutely watch them flourish.

When we nurture our children, they grow up with the confidence to be their true and authentic selves, the selves that God has decreed them to be. They learn to value their own unique traits rather than growing up thinking that they must act in a particular way to gain attention and affection. This means that, as adults, they will be more capable of valuing their time. They will learn to enforce boundaries and say no to things they do not want to do.

How many of us are burnt out because we lack the ability to say no? We think that saying no is nasty or mean because when we were growing up, if someone said no to us, we did not take it as a healthy boundary setting. Instead, we saw it as offensive because we relied heavily on what other people said to boost our sense of self-worth. This is why we have a pandemic of people who have no ability to say no and are unconsciously giving, giving, giving. When we are in a constant state of giving and not filling our own tanks, we teach our children to disregard their own needs and values. Going out of our way to help others is not an issue if we approach it with a full tank. If we operate with an empty tank, resentment will build over time, creating adrenal fatigue and depletion. By the time we recognise this, we may be late in age, and we may regret some of the decisions we made.

By setting healthy boundaries, we not only protect our own self-worth, but teach our children to do the same. Sometimes it is in relation to our own children that these boundaries must be set and enforced. How often do you hear mothers say they "can't go to the bathroom in peace" or "haven't had a chance to eat all day"? This is *not* establishing healthy boundaries and is *not* teaching your children the value of your – or their – worth.

If you are a mother, so much of your life is about giving. It is important to fill up your own cup as well as your family's. After all, you are going to be a much more positive mum if you are well-rested, healthy, and authentically happy. I am not saying that if your child is sick with a fever, you should not stay up catering to them and offering them comfort. Of course you should! You are still a mum, after all, and let us be real – your kids are always going to be your number one priority. What I am talking about is the day to day, the times when you can enforce healthy boundaries with your children so you have the space to breathe, eat, and shower. Doing this will help them learn how to set healthy boundaries themselves and will also instil resilience in them.

Saying things like, "I can't do that right now because I'm going out with friends" or, "In an hour, I'll sit and play with you, but right now I'm reading a book" is an excellent place to start. Your kids need to see you prioritising *you* so they prioritise you and themselves, too.

I tell my children now, "Mum has to leave because she needs time for herself to rest" or, "You need to stay with Dad because Mum is going to go and spend time with her friends. Mum loves you and loves to spend time with you, and she also loves to spend time with her friends." When I started implementing this, initially, my daughter cried every time.

However, nowadays, if she feels that I am distressed or if I have verbalised that I am tired, she will say to me, "Mum, when dad comes home, maybe we can go to Grandma's house while you have a rest." To me, this means that she will also hold this boundary for herself and not do anything for the superficial comfort of others at the cost of her own authentic needs.

Trauma from a Health Perspective

So, you might be thinking, *what does trauma have to do with food?*

Well, my friend, it may surprise you to know that obesity- and diet-related health challenges can be *directly* linked to trauma. This can stem from several different experiences, some of which I will outline below.

Body Image and Our Parents

When it comes to children, a lot of the time, it is monkey see, monkey do. When we shame our own or others' bodies and talk about food negatively in front of children, they mirror this behaviour themselves.

My mother was one of those women who purchased every new weight-loss fad – the lemon detox diet, herbal laxatives, you name it, she tried it – and none of them ever worked. In my eyes, my mother was perfect. In fact, I do not remember her ever being overweight. However, she *perceived* herself as being overweight. So, as a kid growing up, I learned that weight was a bad thing and that being overweight was shameful.

As a result, when I was 18 or 19, I started vomiting every time I ate. I was not overweight by any stretch of the imagination, but I was so fearful of 'getting fat' that I vomited as a preventative measure. I had a lot of shame attached to my body that stemmed from my upbringing. In fact, I remember that no one ever acknowledged my 'heavier' female family members outside of their physical appearances. This intentional vomiting continued for a number of months until I stopped. I was just so sick of activating my gag reflex and worried about the acidity and its impact on my dental health.

We watch our parents' every step and inherit their dysfunctional coping mechanisms as well as their low level of self-worth. It is important that we heal ourselves from this type of trauma so we do not carry it with us and project it onto our children. Imagine if I had not taken the steps to heal my negative body issues! What sort of example would that set for my own children if they had heard me complain about my body or witnessed me vomiting?

Children can be extremely impressionable. So, when Mum says, "I'm ugly," "I'm fat," "I'm no good," her child – who thinks she is perfect in every way possible – is going to think, *If Mum thinks she's so ugly, what does that say about me? I must be ugly too.* It is this ingrained ancestral trauma that continues the chain of low self-worth, which ultimately promotes unhealthy relationships with food.

When you start to speak positively about your image in front of your children, your peers, or your partner, it is important to also align with something that is not a physical attribute, such as intelligence, courage, or patience. This will allow your children to learn that it is not just about being beautiful and we acknowledge them not just because they have beautiful eyes or beautiful hair but because they are intelligent or brave. Our children will then grow up with confidence that is not limited by the perception of physical appearance.

Body Image and the Media

Similarly detrimental, the media can have a lasting negative impact on both adult and child relationships with food and body image through constant displays of what is 'acceptable' and 'attractive'. You know those trashy magazines that litter the supermarket registers, the ones that say celebrity X is too fat and superstar Y is too skinny? Just like they make us feel worthless, they imprint unattainable body standards on our children. Again, this breeds poor physical and mental health.

Back in the late 1990s and early 2000s, the 'desirable' Western female body type was ultra-thin and ultra-blonde. This saw women everywhere starving and bleaching themselves to become the unattainable. Twenty years later, we are seeing a new – and arguably less attainable – trend emerge: the perfect hourglass. This body shape accentuates the chest and buttocks, while the waist remains as thin as possible. Though there are people who are naturally born with thin or hourglass figures, there are far more of us who sit outside these moulds, whether we have smaller hips, bigger thighs, a double chin – the list goes on. Every body shape is beautiful, but the media does not want us to think that. Body diversity is not showcased, leading us to consider ourselves as less-than, unattractive, unlovable. In turn, this breathes billions of dollars into the cosmetics industry.

Everyone is created differently. Of course, genes play a role in shaping our appearances. For example, if your parents have black hair, it is unlikely that yours will be blonde. Or if you have two parents with brown eyes, genetically, chances are your children will also have brown eyes. If your mother has an hourglass figure, it is likely that this may also be your body type, even if you desire to be taller and slimmer. And this is okay. All of it is okay. We must embrace the beauty of difference in an age when the new norm is fillers in the cheeks and lips and tattooed eyebrows. Ironically, we are creating a generation of people who literally look the same but are not related.

Let us talk about ageing for a moment. Since the dawn of time, it has been unacceptable to age. We use Botox on our fine lines and filler in our cheeks. Women as young as 20 are pumping their bodies with chemicals to appear younger and fit the mould of what society deems attractive. Our sense of self-worth is attached to our appearances so if our looks do not meet society's expectations, our self-worth is obliterated.

One day when I was out with my family, I remember staring at a beautiful woman: beautiful skin, eyes, and hair, and beautiful crow's feet around her eyes. As I watched her, I realised how much I missed seeing lines and wrinkles, seeing real people. Instead, I am stuck behind my phone screen, watching people filter their perceived imperfections away. I miss thin lips. I told my sister the other day how beautiful her lips are. She is the only one of the six of us with very thin lips, and I looked at her face in adoration, contrary to the current belief that only full-volume lips are attractive. I looked at the lines on my husband's forehead and realised how handsome it made him. I noticed the beauty of the regrowth of my cousin's brows. I saw beauty in places and in people where it was no longer acknowledged, according to society's standards. I looked at the scar on my own face, at my beauty spots, and remembered how unique they are to me. These things that once made me so conscious of my body, I now viewed as beauty.

Toxic Beauty

How bizarre is it that our government has banned cannabis, and numerous other beneficial foods and plants, but allows Botox? Botox is actually a very dangerous toxin. It is made from botulinum bacteria, which is then injected into the muscle. When administered correctly, it is not *usually* harmful, though it is technically a poison that acts by paralysing the muscle temporarily. The effects of Botox wear off once the body acknowledges that there is a toxin in it and formulates a way to release it. My theory on the human body's relationship with this toxin is that people who are unhealthy or whose livers may not be functioning optimally notice that their Botox lasts longer. The healthier a person is, the less time the effects of Botox last. Botox does not delay the ageing process; rather, it temporarily masks it. From what I have witnessed, long-term use will cause more ageing of the skin unless you continuously use Botox because as the skin stretches a certain way and stays in that position until the toxin wears off, the muscular strength is compromised.

Fillers are in the same category. Currently, there is not a great deal of information about the long-term side effects of filler. However, we do know that whether they are made from hydrochloric acid or synthetic materials, fillers may cause complications, such as muscle weakness, bruising, and swelling, for patients down the track.[67] Regardless, we ignore the potential physical and psychological side effects of long-term filler and Botox use for the sake of our external satiety. Even if it were safe, the problem here is not the filler; it is the extent to which we are willing to change our authentic physical self for external satiation and validation.

Due to being brought up in a superficial fashion, we use toxins to prevent wrinkles, as opposed to accepting that the ageing process is natural. If God blesses us with a long life, we should be grateful that we have lived to an age where we wrinkle and sag! The more we rely on unnatural solutions, the more likely our children are to feel the pressure to do the same, again, promoting the perpetual cycle of low self-esteem and body image.

Recently, I caught up with one of my girlfriends who had extremely large, fake lashes on. She told me that she grew up with a mum who thought self-care was about lathering your face in make-up, wearing fake lashes, and getting your lips done. She thought you had to look beautiful, which is why, as a woman in her thirties, my friend felt pressured to wear false lashes. She wanted to live up to her own mother's standards.

The only way to *really* delay superficial ageing is to ensure that we are eating antioxidant- and collagen-rich foods, staying hydrated, reducing exposure to harmful chemicals, such as those in some food and cigarettes, exercising, and making sure the detox pathways in the body are constantly cleansing so free radicals do not create damage. That is what is going to keep your skin looking younger, not an army of people prodding your face with needles!

Food and Trauma

Do you remember when you were a child and your parents made you finish everything on your plate because you had to eat what you were given, and the kids in Africa were starving? Maybe you make these sorts of comments to your own kids. Well, I hate to break it to you, but this is one *incredibly* common example of behaviour that can lead to food trauma.

Encouraging children to eat everything on their plate is not as harmless as it may seem. By encouraging children to eat past fullness, you are:

A. Disconnecting them from their ability to acknowledge satiety

B. Promoting emotional relationships with food, the same ones that perhaps you have.

Let me explain. Children obey their parents out of fear, guilt, and a desire to please. When parents reward or punish children for finishing – or not finishing – a meal, they attach these emotions to food. For example, if a child is forced to sit at the table until they have eaten everything on their plate, they will be fearful of not finishing food in the future, learning not to trust their physical feelings of satiation. Conversely, if a child receives praise for eating past fullness, they will associate overeating with positive outcomes (praise) and learn to attach happy feelings to eating to excess.

These emotions disconnect the child from their intuitive gut. As we grow older, this translates to an emotional and unhealthy relationship with food, where it becomes a means of contentment. Whether we have a void that can be attributed to a lack of self-love, a lack of self-worth, or a lack of a sense of belonging, we turn to food because it momentarily comforts us and makes us feel better. We then experience feelings of guilt and shame because we have consumed foods in amounts that we intuitively know are unbeneficial.

When a child is repetitively forced to keep eating, they learn to ignore their body's signals that tell them they are full. This affects their natural appetite later in life. They do not know when to stop, which can lead to a plethora of physical problems (obesity, type 2 diabetes, cardiovascular disease) and psychological problems (disordered eating, depression, anxiety). While encouraging a child to eat may seem harmless and, in essence, caring, it can actually create problems with their relationship with food and cause the very trauma we wish to avoid. Although our parents did not intend for us to become people who eat for reward, here we are, decades later, addicted to food and using it for emotional comfort.

We should honour our satiation signals. In the life of the Prophet (PBUH), he was never seen eating until he was full, and his companions commented that he had no belly before he passed, so he was not overweight.

How We Negatively Shape a Child's Self-Esteem

As we now know, the negative information we receive about food as children can develop into body issues later in life. In addition to what we have already discussed, there are many other seemingly inconsequential ways we can negatively shape a child's self-esteem.

1. ATTACHING 'GOOD' AND 'BAD' LABELS TO FOOD

This is a tricky one. Of course, you want your child to eat high-quality foods, so you tell them which are good and which are not. You might even lure your child to eat their carrots, a 'good' food, with the incentive of ice cream, a 'treat'. I hate to break it to you, but this breeds problems for your child, as they begin to attach their worth to the foods they consume: "I ate bad food, therefore I am bad."

Instead, it is important to neutralise the way we talk about food. Instead of referring to foods as 'good' and 'bad', try referring to traditionally healthy foods as 'nutritious' and 'delicious', and stereotypically unhealthy foods as 'pleasurable' and 'comforting'. When we remove the stigma from certain foods, we detach feelings of shame, guilt, and loathing. This can help us lead healthier lives, both physically and mentally.

How often have you succumbed to temptation by eating 'bad' food? I am guessing *many times*. But so have I, and I continue to do so. There is, of course, nothing wrong with this. However, if we attach negativity to that food, we will immediately feel ashamed after we consume it. For some, it can ruin their entire day. Additionally, when we eat foods that we consider bad, we can ultimately end up consuming *more*. We think, Oh well, *I've gone and done it now* when we snack on a bowl of ice cream. *I may as well finish off the tub!*

Part of the problem is that we use food to fill the void that should hold spiritual light. At a time when materialism and physical appearance has become profoundly important, it is no surprise that our lack of spiritual connection has led to us filling that void with the consumption of food.

2. RESTRICTING OR PROHIBITING CERTAIN FOODS

The more limits we put on certain food, the more desirable they become. When I was a kid, my parents did not let us have soft drinks. We were never allowed Coke and never allowed to go to McDonalds. No surprise, we grew up *resenting* those rules. However, as our parents had explained the 'why' behind the no, it enabled us to make more empowered decisions, as opposed to us stopping something temporarily from fear of authority. We learned to avoid those foods because there was a good, sound, logical reason not to consume them.

Now, I am not saying that parents should completely neglect the good nutrition of their children. After all, we each carry the responsibility to keep our kids well-fed, fit, and healthy. However, it is undeniable that the more you forbid something, the more enticing it becomes. The minute you detach emotion from food is the same minute it comes off its pedestal. This is true for everyone, but especially for children. Therefore, instead of the current approaches we use to prevent our children from eating food that may cause harm to their bodies, explaining to them in a way that they understand and giving them some level of autonomy, power, and confidence to make the decision themselves will lead to little humans who are well-equipped to make favourable food choices.

I was an absolute anti-sugar mum when my daughter was one. She was vegan until she was two because I was vegan, and I would not allow her to have any foods I thought were unhealthy. However, as she grew older, I started attaching reason to my decisions. "We can't have this because it has a chemical in it that's bad for the body." This is what I would say to my three-year-old. You do not need to give all the details. When young, they do not need to know what an older child may want to know. They just want boundaries set in a respectful – rather than authoritarian – way.

When my daughter was six, we would enter the grocery store, and she would pick up something that she was attracted to because of the packaging, bringing it to me to read. "Mum, do these ingredients contain sugar?" she would ask. "Are there any chemicals in here?" My six year old was not necessarily more intelligent than any other six year old. However, from a very young age, I allowed her a level of autonomy over her own body so she would feel empowered to make her own decisions. Although, in essence, they were rhetorical decisions. I knew that, the majority of the time, she would not be consuming food labelled as having large amounts of sugar or undesirable chemicals.

Other food boundaries we have set include ingredients such as cochineal, which is literally red bugs that are used to colour some foods and drinks. When we empower our children to understand the information we provide and make their own informed decisions, we do not need to rely on authoritarianism and angst to create boundaries they may not even comprehend.

To be completely honest, I do not want my kids to eat hot chips because, usually when purchased out, they are just toxic vegetable oils with a starchy vegetable that is full of sugars. But, once in a while, if they ask me for hot chips, I am going to get them for them. I am not going to make them miss out and resent me and the food I cook. That would only make them want hot chips more, and when they finally do get them, they would be more likely to binge. They might even experience feelings of shame after eating them because I told them "no" their entire lives. Rather than prohibiting specific foods, try explaining their contents and the effect they have on the human body. Do this in a neutral way and let your child know that it is ultimately up to them to decide what goes into their bodies. How much detail you provide will depend on the maturity of the child.

For example, when it comes to my kids – who are still quite young – I explain to them in basic terms what chemicals are, when they are found in foods, and how they can affect the human body. Hence, when they are confronted with a food choice, they can make an informed and autonomous decision about whether or not they want to consume that food. Whatever decision they make receives a neutral reaction.

For example, my daughter and I were out, and she wanted a lollipop. We spoke about how this lollipop was full of sugar and chemicals and what it meant for her health. She said she still felt like having a lick. Of course, I gave her my permission and said, "You can lick the lollipop until you decide to stop."

She started to lick, continuing for the next couple of minutes, and then handed me the lollipop. "Here you go, Mum," she said. "I don't like sugar. I don't want to finish this lollipop anymore." Consciously, my daughter listened to her body and made a healthy decision. It is not always a happy ending, though. Sometimes she wants to eat something she knows is unhealthy, which is okay. How many times have you eaten rubbish, knowing it will not serve you and having better comprehension around health than a five year old? Many times, just like me.

On another occasion, we walked into a dessert store, and she saw a massive chocolate lollipop with hundreds and thousands all over it. I said to her, "Let's read the ingredients," to which she agreed. "Look," I said, "this lollipop has a lot of chemicals. Look at all the numbers." She understands that numbers generally mean chemicals. "Do you think we should be eating this?" I asked.

"But I really feel like it," she said.

"Okay," I said. "I'm going to buy it, and you can have as much as you like. When you no longer want to eat it, you can throw it in the bin."

We made the purchase, and my daughter took a couple of bites. After that, she threw it out. If I had not allowed her to have that experience, she may then have purchased it behind my back with someone who may not have explained the effects that those chemicals could have on her body. Or she may internalise resentment or an additional desire for things she cannot have. As a result, there may not be a conscious awareness associated with making that decision. Our goal is to raise conscious little humans to the best of our ability, and this is not going to happen until we become a nation of people who turn food packages around and read the labels. We must examine the ingredients, understand their effects on our bodies, and make informed decisions to eat or avoid particular foods based on self-love and self-worth.

3. REMOVING CHILDREN'S AUTONOMY AROUND FOOD

As I mentioned earlier, giving your child the autonomy to decide what to put into their body – within boundaries, of course – will give them the tools to make healthier choices. When a child is young, the only autonomy they have relates to food and sleep. They do not have control over much else in their lives – the adults decide everything. When we take that control from them, they may act out in other areas.

I noticed this in my own child. When I was more restrictive in my approach to food, my daughter began making unconscious behavioural changes. For example, she started overreacting to minor things and showed a low level of patience that she had not before. When I eased my approach and gave her back some control, she felt more liberated, and the resistance melted away.

You need to give your child some level of autonomy to create resilience in them, rather than just oppressing them with power and discipline. Doing this equips them with the strength and ability to make conscious decisions as they grow. The more you speak to them in healthy adult conversation, the more resilient and intelligent they become. When we invest time and energy in educating our children, we help facilitate a healthy relationship with food.

This is also the benchmark in Islam. There is no coercion in religion; there is no force. We cannot become Muslims under duress. However, we also know that nothing is without consequence. There are consequences to every decision we make in our lives. We can feed our children whatever we want as long as we are conscious of the short- and long-term impact the food is going to have on them.

4. ATTACHING MEANING WHERE NONE EXISTS

It is not what happens to us but how we respond that matters.

Our life experiences influence how we respond to future situations. Everyone will experience hurt, loss, fear, grief, and anger in their lives. These experiences and feelings mould us – for better or worse – into who we are today. We can either choose to heal and learn from these experiences, or we can let them drag us down and influence our future thoughts and behaviours in negative ways.

Often, those who do not heal from life experiences project their unresolved traumas onto others. This may come in the form of attaching meaning to words, behaviours, or situations where none exists or at least where the meaning is not what they think it is. Therefore, you can say the same thing using the same words in the same tone to two different people and receive two different reactions. Each person projects their unhealed traumas onto you via their reaction to your statement, and each has their own filters that they use when they translate what you are saying to them.

For example, if you say, "Don't eat that chocolate bar" to a child who has been constantly belittled about their weight, that child is going to be flooded with shameful thoughts around that comment based on how they already feel about themselves. So, they may translate what you said to mean: "You're ugly." "You're greedy." Or, "You're worthless." Their past experiences – mainly being bullied about their weight – activate certain filters. In their mind, any comment that relates to food is an attack on them and their body.

Now, when you say the same thing to a child who has not been bullied about their weight but has been educated about healthy eating, they will not attach the same meaning or experience feelings of shame. Instead, for this second child, the very same comment may be taken at surface value as caring, as the child knows it is not healthy to eat that bar and, thus, acknowledges that whoever has made the comment has done so from a place of love. They understand that you have a point – a point that is indeed both valid and healthy.

Let us all aspire to be great influences on our children by resolving our own trauma so we do not display damaging behaviour to them. By healing ourselves, we can better guide our children through their own experiences of hurt and healing, rather than contributing to them.

Awareness is Key

In everything, awareness is key. Once we understand something objectively, rather than through a subjective lens tainted by trauma, we are more able to make conscious decisions about it.

Let us take breast implants, for example. Implants can act as a solution to years of insecurity, a remedy for uneven tissue, or an answer to an unwanted mastectomy. There are many reasons why people undergo this surgery, and all are valid. I hold no judgement.

Cultural expectations in the 21st century dictate that women with fuller breasts are more appealing. We must acknowledge the role that trauma – caused by our parents, the media, and society more generally – plays regarding this expectation. It is the trauma that says we must look a certain way to be considered attractive. If we remove that trauma and focus entirely on the health implications associated with breast implants, such as autoimmune illnesses, it becomes less likely that we would subject our bodies to that kind of risk simply to fit in with societal beauty standards.[68]

Is this not what we are doing when we educate and empower our children with knowledge and information around food? If we did this with children who later opted for breast implants as adults to look better, perhaps they would have had a better chance of being comfortable and happy in their own skin.

When we start to peel back the layers of our trauma, we begin to see things with clarity and objectivity. We see things for how they really are, rather than how we have been conditioned to view or translate them through the lenses created by our upbringing.

We each need to take the time to truly become aware of our hidden traumas so we may start to heal them and lead healthier lives. Once we acknowledge the existence of our trauma, which every single one of us has, we can make more conscious decisions for our health, with our minds no longer clouded by predetermined beliefs. Therefore, we have no need for the attachment of the external synthetic pleasures.

The Intersection of Food and Faith

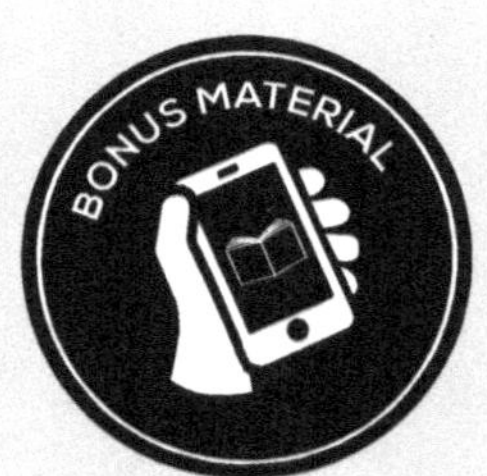

Julide is sharing more
in her BONUS CONTENT.

Scan the QR code or visit
www.julideturkernw.com/product/
one-third-of-your-stomach/bonus-content
to access additional content.

CHAPTER FIVE

INTRODUCTION TO FOOD: A BRIEF OVERVIEW OF THE EFFECTS OF FOOD ON THE BODY

"Do not kill your hearts by eating and drinking too much. For the heart is like a sown field: over-irrigation causes the seed to rot."
– Ibn Sina (Avicenna)

Food is Medicine (or Poison)

I find it mind-blowing that the first sin committed by Adam involved his mouth: he ate the forbidden fruit in heaven. It is especially astounding when we know that the soul comes out of the mouth when we die. When we marry these spiritual signs with the physical – for example, disease starts in the mouth – the oral cavity either provides the opportunity for digestion and the inhibition of pathogenic growth or, on the contrary, causes further illnesses throughout the body. As a matter of fact, each tooth is connected to an organ through the nervous system; this is covered thoroughly in dental neurobiology.[69] Thus, in a holistic paradigm, the tooth experiencing an issue is not seen just as a decaying tooth but also as a sign of an unwell organ.

Food can either heal us from a state of disease or act as a slow poison. What we put into our bodies determines our health. If you overfill your body with poor food, it can only respond with sickness and pain.

The issue is that, in our fast-paced lifestyles, just as we expect healing to come in a moment, we expect something detrimental to happen quickly, too. What I mean by this is that when you have a cup of soda you assume that if there is no immediate symptom, there is no issue to worry about. However, poisons accumulate in body tissue, and they certainly do cause issues but not always immediately. They can be especially problematic if detoxification is not achieved, which I will speak about more in the chapter on fasting.

According to Islamic scholar Ibn al-Qayyim, there is but one physical consequence of overconsumption: disease. He tells us that most illnesses are driven by gorging on foods and, to preserve the body, we must eat a balanced diet, allowing time to digest properly before we consume again.

In his book, *Zad al-Ma'ad* (translated as *Provisions for the Hereafter*), Ibn al-Qayyim describes illness as follows: "Illnesses are of two types. Material illnesses arise from an increase of matter that comes to a point of excess in the body where it harms its natural functions. **And these are the majority of illnesses**."[70] What Ibn al-Qayyim means is that diseases are mostly, if not completely, caused by consuming more food before the food taken previously has been properly digested, which includes eating in excess of the amount needed by the body, taking in food that is of little nutritional value and is slow to digest, and indulging in different foods that are complex in their composition. When a human being fills his belly with these foods and it becomes a habit, they cause him various diseases, some of which come to an end slowly, and some swiftly. When he is **moderate in his eating** and takes only as much food as he needs, **keeping a balance of quantity and quality**, the body benefits more from this than it does from a large amount of food.

When reading this, we need to consider the word 'disease' in its broadest sense. For example, overeating might make us feel sluggish, drowsy, and uncomfortable. Some people may also experience gastrointestinal issues, like irregular bowel movements, bloating, gas, and reflux. Though these issues may not be strictly branded diseases and instead labelled symptoms in the Western medical sense, they are included within Ibn al-Qayyim's elucidation of material illness caused by food, as they are symptoms that if not immediately addressed and corrected will inevitably lead to illness over time.

Of course, what Ibn al-Qayyim really warns of are the long-term effects of habitually eating too much, or eating the wrong type of, food. For, "It is when overeating becomes sustained over long periods that it becomes a health risk."[71] When we regularly consume food of poor quality or in excessive quantities, we experience severer symptoms than those listed earlier. For example, eating again prior to digestion means that we consume more calories than our bodies need and we are mixing foods that are not supposed to be combined. As a result, we make digestion difficult, and the body must divert more energy to the digestive process rather than conserving it for healing and repair. This can cause weight gain and obesity, which can lead to cardiovascular disease, cancer, hypertension, and type 2 diabetes.[72] In fact, when physician of the Arabs, Harith ibn Kalada, was asked what the disease was, he replied, "The introduction of food on top of food before it has been digested."[73]

Ideal Food Combinations

The types of food we consume and allow to mix can exacerbate the symptoms of bloating, indigestion, and reflux. Thus, food combining is an important art to consider. In Islam, we look at this from the paradigm of the Prophet's (PBUH) teachings. He suggests that dry foods should be mixed with wet to obtain some liquid consistency for the ease of digestion, and foods that are high in calories, such as dates, must be combined with something that will regulate the glycaemic index, such as milk, so the food does not immediately cause an imbalance in blood glucose levels. Yes, this wisdom existed way before there was any solid information or research on food combining.

Do you ever wonder why, as Muslims, we are told to break our fast with either salt, dates, or water? Dates are high in sugar. Taken alone and immediately, they raise blood sugar, which is exactly what is needed after being in a state of hunger for more than ten hours. Salt does something similar: the minerals wake the body up, and the cells work like a battery. I am not talking about iodine-added or regular table salt, which is highly refined and stripped of its minerals. I am referring to salt in its natural state, for example, Celtic salt. Finally, water increases the movement of blood and lymph, thus creating an immediate shift in energy levels. Breaking fast in this way is also in Hadith: "The Messenger of Allah (PBUH) used to break his fast with fresh dates before praying. If there were no fresh dates, then with dried dates, and if there were no dried dates, then with a few sips of water."[74]

Modern science supports the idea that the combination of foods consumed affects health, as different foods undergo different digestive processes. Thus, when food combination is done correctly, we absorb the correct sequence of amino acids to create protein and repair damaged tissue. In contrast, if we do not combine our foods properly, we can develop nutrient imbalances, amino acid deficiencies – which can cause issues with tissue repair – and increased acidity.[75]

In the 21st century, combining foods correctly has become extremely challenging, as many fruits and vegetables are hybrid, so they are not in the authentic nutritional forms that God intended. Instead, they are man-made genetic compositions that boost revenue by being easier to grow in unfavourable climates and better tasting.

In our community, this is one of the most common misconceptions about food. We assume that if something is organic, it is not hybrid. However, you can have a hybrid seed and grow it organically. So, let us go to square one. Hybrid foods are defined as those that are crossbred to create produce that maximises desirable traits. Desired traits may include increased durability, production yield, size of the fruit or vegetable, and improved taste.

So, are hybrid foods genetically modified? No, they are not: "GMO seeds are produced by genetic engineering, altering the genetic material of an organism, whereas hybrid seeds are produced by crossbreeding of two varieties through artificial mating."[76]

As Muslims, we have an innate connection to the philosophy that everything that is created by God is already perfect. We are not in a place to modify it or change it in any way.

In a seminar conducted by Islamic scholars in Kuwait in 1998, it was concluded that there was no sound Islamic law that prohibited the use of genetically modified foods based on their potential negative effects on humans and the environment. Further to this, the Indonesian Scholars Council, in 2003, released an Islamic statement allowing the use and consumption of genetically modified products for their people.[77] On the other hand, some scholars are of the view that GMO foods are not permissible under Islamic law due to altering things that should only exist in the way God created and intended them to be, not allowing for any change, which includes creating man-made hybrids and performing genetic modification.

Some suggest that the opposition to GMO is based on the philosophy that God created everything in perfection and that man has no right to manipulate. If he does, potentially, more harm than benefit can come from it in the long run, and there are too many unknowns to be able to consider the advantage versus disadvantage from an Islamic jurisprudence perspective.

I hold the latter opinion: what God has made is unique and perfect as is, and no modification is essential, especially when you consider that modification or hybridisation generally occurs for the pleasure of the consumer, often by enhancing flavours, and to fill the pockets of company owners. Even when one justifies the use of GMOs to, say, allow the crop to withstand a colder climate, we have to go back to rooting ourselves in ethics and ask why, for example, there is climate change as a result of what we have created with our own hands and why a particular crop is not growing in a particular soil. It may not be fit for that soil. The crop may have been imported from another country, so the benefit of having it may not necessarily outweigh the disadvantage of not eating it.

The matter must be considered from an environmental, socio political, spiritual, and religious perspective. We cannot just say it is okay because we need the fruit to taste sweeter or we need to reap more produce with the same seed. Islam is a way of life; it is not a list of rules; it is not a to-do list full of yeses and noes. There are many things left in the grey, which means we need to go back to embodying the lifestyle of the Prophet (PBUH) and seeing if the desired outcome aligns with the philosophy of Islam. We are the vicegerents of the Earth, but that does not mean we trot on it in disregard. It means we protect everything living on it, from the bees, to the plants that grow, to the quality of the soil.

Eating in excess is also frowned upon in other religions, such as Christianity. Gluttony is one of the seven deadly sins, right? Eating more than you need does a lot to dysregulate homeostasis in the body. So much more energy is required to break down that food; so much work needs to be done by the liver to break it down, and we end up using more vitamins and bacteria to assist in this process. Therefore, it is literally a waste of our vital and important energy reserves that, quite frankly, we are already low on as it is in a world laced with chemicals: in our food, in our water, in our skies, and in the hybrid foods that we eat, day in, and day out.

Snacking is one of the most common things we all do that is so against our fitrah, which is Arabic for 'nature' or 'innate needs'. There are so many issues with snacking, but I will list only some. The more we eat, the more the body has to make stomach acid, release digestive enzymes, and use up energy for the constant breakdown and digestive processes. We risk our teeth to caries and decay earlier, especially in our children, because we are left with loads of simple, refined sugars and carbs that our oral microbiome has to deal with.[78]

Snacking also hinders the body's ability to break down and absorb the prior food consumed, which means that not only are we not absorbing the minerals and vitamins that are vital for every single cellular process in the body, but we are also putting more work on the vital organs and rushing them to ageing and losing the ability to work effectively.

Have you ever considered why people are diagnosed with high stomach acid or hyperchlorhydria? It is a very common phenomenon nowadays, and one cause may be the excessive consumption of meat and its inability to properly combine with vegetables and leafy greens. This causes the stomach to make more acid to break down the excessive amounts of animal protein, which can lead to hyperacidity symptoms.[79] This is all in the literature, by the way, and has been for decades.

When we look at consuming meat, we have the same blind man approach because when we see meat, we only see protein. We do not see the cholesterol and the hormones, such as estrogen and testosterone. We do not see the antibiotics that end up stored in the animal's fat, and so on. We only see 'protein' and 'healthy protein' in lean meats, which is, again, a linear view of a complex image. There are many references to reducing the consumption of meat in Islamic history. As a matter of fact, in the Maliki school of thought, only the rich women were allowed to consume meat and were limited to consuming it once a week – because we knew the spiritual chaos excess meat could lead to.

Coming back to the stomach acid – do you see how one-eyed it is? We only see one perspective. We do not view eating meat holistically. When we consume animal proteins too often – for example, every day or multiple times per day – our bodies break down these proteins by increasing the acidity in the stomach. This is also the way to ensure that no bacteria or other microbes remain and to prevent them from causing an imbalance in the body. However, when we consume meat excessively and, thus, then trigger excess stomach acid, we see our doctor and get prescribed an antacid. When we take antacid and reduce the amount of acid made by the stomach, we not only make it harder to break down proteins because now the stomach acid is too low, but we also create other issues, such as a predisposition to bacterial and fungal infections, as the stomach acid may not be the right calibre to denature and kill off these pathogens. So, the treatment of the symptom is rarely the solution to the actual disease.

Through our functional medicine model, we acknowledge that as opposed to rejecting the body's innate intelligence in overproducing stomach acid to break down excess protein, it would be wiser and more in alignment with the body's innate functionality to reduce or remove the cause of the excess production In this example, it is the excess consumption of meat.

The benefit of stomach acid is that it is the 'checkpoint' for many protozoa, parasites, parasitic eggs, larva, and the like coming into the stomach. The acid kills off any foreign microorganism that should not be there and when we suppress this function, it cannot complete this task well. Once again, we are looking at the elephant from one man's view as opposed to accepting it in its entirety.

Food with low nutritional value is another massive issue. We consume packaged everything that is overly processed and then fortified because the very method of processing these foods takes away the nutrition, potentially creating nutritional deficiencies. For example, have you ever wondered why we have iodised salt? Iodised salt is when the mineral iodine is added into our regular table salt. In Australia, we add it due to an epidemic of low thyroid function, which the literature blames on a widespread deficiency in iodine.[80] We do not get iodine naturally in table salt because we bleach the salt after harvesting, removing many of the minerals it began with. So, we are left with only two minerals: sodium and chloride – and iodine, of course, once we have added it back in.

The reality is that, one day, man will come to understand that the limited abilities God has blessed us with means that we will continue to make immense mistakes in our food chain. It will always be a decade or two after we have caused some serious collateral damage that we wake up and say, "Oh, science was wrong."

Let us now explore another important point Ibn Qayyim mentioned: the incorrect combining of food, or as he says, "… indulging in different foods which are complex in their composition."[81] Meat is a complex food to digest, so is dairy, by the way. I also see it as eating things that are not supposed to be eaten together or are eaten close together from a time line perspective, which comes back to eating again prior to digesting the previous meal. Proper food combining involves the consumption of grains with legumes, grains with seeds, nuts and seeds with vegetables, and animal-based proteins with vegetables. The typical meal of a burger, chips, and bottle of soft drink is a recipe for wreaking havoc on stomach acidity levels, reducing our ability to break down foods that must travel to every cell in the body to perform hundreds of enzymatic reactions crucial to our survival.

Sugar, in and of itself, is an antinutrient. So, we may already be deficient in vitamins and minerals in our bodies; then we have this foodstuff coming in called sugar that is depleting our already low vitamin levels, while the vitamins aid in its elimination process, further fatiguing organs, such as the liver.[82]

So, why should we not have a starch, like bread or potato chips, with a meat-based protein, like a beef patty? Because there is a theory that protein and starches require different environments for digestion. According to some theorists, the body cannot supply the two different environments simultaneously, so its ability to break down each food type is compromised. For this reason, when we have a barbeque, we have to have an acidic drink with it because we have eaten so much bread and meat that the stomach struggles to disintegrate it all. Unconsciously, we consume something to temporarily aid with the lack of acid production.

The other side to this is that breaking down improperly combined food leads to excessive energy expenditure. Therefore, less energy is left over for cellular repair and exosome detoxification. As Ibn Qayyim says, we have compromised our healing and health by eating this way.[83] How does this translate to our spiritual calibre? Perhaps the excess wind means we cannot keep our ablution, which needs to be redone every time we use the bathroom, break wind, have sexual intercourse, or vomit. Then we resent the prayer because we need to perform ablution again, which takes more time, so we compromise the time we invest in prayer because we have already lost five minutes performing our ablution. Or the lack of the body's ability to heal and repair means that we wake up for morning prayer with low energy and are not spiritually and physically present. We may forget what we want to pray for, and, all of a sudden, prayer is nothing more than a number of robotic movements, a far stretch from its original intention.

Improper food combining also contributes to weight gain. Even though we do not need more calories, we are nutritionally deprived, and the signal our body gives us to eat more is actually a signal to say that the cells are starving for nutrition, but we recognise this as hunger. As a result, we eat that extra burger or another spoonful of white rice, and the cycle continues. No one can say that it does not physically impede their daily prayers or the task of living life as a conscious human being. The discomfort causes us to have a shorter fuse with our children and to need more sleep, reducing our quality of life. We become so invested in our own physical issues that we have just enough energy to survive each day, not even to thrive. We are so entrapped in our own problems that we have no time, energy, or ability to do anything for anyone else, which creates a disconnected community of people who are alive, but that is all that they are – alive.

Have you ever wondered why religion puts such a large emphasis on food? Why the Hadiths mention food all the time? Why the Qur'an speaks of it? Why so many of our renowned scholars have written about it? Why preventative medicine involves how we eat and how we live our lives? This is because the foods we eat create our thoughts and our mental health. Neurotransmitters, which are chemical messengers of the brain, are mostly made in the small intestine. So, feeling happy, or sad, or angry, or excited, or motivated largely involves the food we eat. Thus, Islam sees a very prominent and strong relationship between the food we eat and our spiritual and mental states.

Water and Food

Drinking without food is a huge problem as well. There is a theory that water impedes the digestive process by combining more liquid than the stomach can tolerate. As a result, we dilute nutrition and disturb the process of peristalsis. This may be why, Islamically, we are encouraged to keep our meal separate from our food. Instead, we have a wet and dry meal to ensure it is moist enough for peristalsis and movement but not so wet that it inhibits the digestive process, dilutes the food, and expands the stomach. The Prophet (PBUH) appreciated this fact, as referenced numerous times throughout the Hadith: "The Apostle of Allah (SAW) came out from the valley of a mountain where he had eased himself. There were some dried dates on a shield before us. We called him and he ate with us. He did not touch the water."[84]

Chemicals of the Brain

Chemicals that control the brain and neurological functions are, in fact, not made in the brain. They are largely made in the gastrointestinal tract. Around 90 percent of serotonin – a chemical labelled the 'happiness hormone' – is manufactured in the small intestine.[85] As a matter of fact, a large proportion of all stress and sex hormones are made in the gut and not just in the brain, adrenal glands, and reproductive organs. Therefore, what we eat has a direct impact on how our brain functions. This is a profound reason why Islam puts so much emphasis on preventative medicine and teaching us not just what to eat, but how to eat, how much to eat, and even when to eat. While we are looking for the next fad diet as the solution to our problems, the answers are already right there in ancient wisdom.

To take it a step further, serotonin is a precursor for melatonin, which is a sleep hormone. Without it, we cannot fall or stay asleep properly. Many people who suffer from digestive compromise also suffer from insomnia because when their body cannot make serotonin, it is unable to manufacture melatonin, resulting in symptoms and illnesses caused by lack of sleep. Sleep is super important when it comes to our ability to detoxify, rest, and recuperate.

Importance of Consuming Wholesome Food

The Qur'an advises us, **"Ye People, eat of what is on earth, lawful and wholesome"** (2:168).

In the time of the Prophet (PBUH), foods were mostly pure, in that nothing was chemically sprayed. Therefore, everything was organic. There were no hybrid foods, and people mostly ate in season, ate what was fresh and not frozen, ate only to their fill, and overconsumption and obesity were rare. However, so much has changed that it makes it harder for us to acknowledge what is permissible and what is not, as it is not as black and white as it was 1400 years ago.

Many people have difficulty understanding what 'whole' foods are because so few people actually eat them. As few as two hundred years ago, everyone consumed wholefoods because processed foods were not an option. Wholefoods are foods that are not packaged, not modified, not grown out of season, not extensively sprayed. They are fruits, grains and vegetables that are the way God intended them to be. A wholefood is a food that has retained its original constituents.

So many man-made errors occur when we attempt to replicate nature. This may be why the Qur'an advises against changing the natural form of anything. For example, pasteurisation does a lot to prevent disease, which is especially important now because of our cattle's poor quality of life. Their milk's microbiome is distorted, which is one reason why, in factory farming, we have to pasteurise milk. Otherwise, we will get sick (more on this in the chapter on halal and tayyib). When we pasteurise, we kill off all the beneficial microbiome that we would otherwise get from milk. Then, to make up for it, we artificially add it at the end in amounts and strains that we think are best, which are far from the original healthy quality and quantities that God intended.

We add folate to bread because the naturally occurring folate in it is much less than what it would have been had we kept it in its natural form. To recreate a 'nutritious' food, we must put the folate back in, which is completely out of synchronicity with nature and, thus, God.

The only way we can guarantee we are getting all of our nutrients is to get them from wholefoods. Attempting to build our health any other way is pseudoscientific. We acknowledge that science is ever-changing, so, as much as we give it the benefit of the doubt, we should also take it with a grain of salt. Furthermore, it does not make sense to eat devitalised foods and then spend time and money buying vitamins and supplements and following various health programs to mitigate the damage done to the body. We eat low-quality diets and try to compensate by taking pills and although some benefits cannot be dismissed, the disadvantages are higher.

The Qur'an also advises us to, **"Eat of the good things We have provided for your sustenance, but commit no excess therein"** (20:81).

The Prophet (PBUH) was known to eat fruits and vegetables grown in the region in which he lived and in season.[86] This is a significant statement on how Islam emphasises the importance of eating in season. Before I studied nutrition at university, I did not even know which fruits and vegetables were grown in which season. Living in Australia and having access to all foods all the time, no one second-guesses eating a strawberry in winter.

Because we have access to all fruits and vegetables year-round, few people understand nature's innate intelligence regarding why onions grow in autumn and winter. The answer is that they support the immune system and detox pathways. At various times, our cells cleanse and shed accumulated toxins. The same cleansing occurs in everything around us. For example, trees lose their leaves, but we do not label them sick for doing so. We acknowledge that their genetic imprint compels them to cleanse and develop new leaves that are conducive to its health. In the same way, we sometimes get sick during autumn and winter, but not always due to exposure to a bug. We are programmed by God to detoxify in alignment with nature, as accumulating toxins create the foundations for a shorter life span and chronic illnesses in the future.

So, what about summer and spring? Berries are abundant in these seasons because they are high in nutrients that benefit the cells and promote their proper function. This perfectly aligns with the belief that God designed the growth of foods to match our innate needs, as He is the one who knows man better than man knows himself.

Filling One Third of Our Stomachs

Another Hadith I will mention again is that of Al-Miqdad: "The son of Adam cannot fill a vessel worse than his stomach, as it is enough for him to take a few bites to straighten his back. If he cannot do it, then he may fill it with a third of his food, a third of his drink, and a third of his breath."[87] This sets a benchmark for us in terms of the upper and lower limits of what we should eat. All it takes is a few bites of food for us to be satiated. However, if that is intolerable, we may eat to our fill but *only* if the food fills no more than one third of the stomach. Considering the modern state of food, filling one third of our stomachs does not necessarily provide the satiation it would have 1400 years ago.

This Hadith also demonstrates the importance of water. Many of us do not drink enough or know how much is required. The Hadith tells us that we should drink the same volume as we eat, meaning that water intake is just as important as food. From a scientific perspective, the hormone ghrelin, which signals hunger to the brain, also indicates thirst. So, if you are someone who does not drink much water but regularly feels hungry, there is a possibility that your body is actually telling you it is dehydrated and water is needed.

Although these guidelines were recorded thousands of years ago, they continue to hold up against modern science. In fact, a recent study conducted by the National Institute of Health (NIH) found that people who ate an ultra-processed diet ingested more calories and gained more weight than those who consumed a diet that was minimally processed.[88] In the study, 20 participants were each given a processed and unprocessed diet for 14 days. Although both diets "were matched for presented calories, sugar, fat, fibre, and micronutrients," each participant consumed approximately 500 more calories per day when on the processed diet, which led to an increase in weight.

Manufacturing Food Addiction

When we eat bad food, we tend to *overeat* bad food. The combination of chemicals, salts, and fats in processed meals makes it hard for us to say no to one more bite, snack, or serving. In fact, junk food is purposely built that way. Unfortunately, the other truth is that chemical engineers and food scientists are constantly inventing flavours and additives to make food more addictive so we keep coming back for more – even after we swore it would be our last bite!

Think about MSG (monosodium glutamate), a food additive commonly found in takeaway, processed, and pre-packaged meals. This is a chemical that not only enhances the flavour of food, making your pack of potato crisps that much harder to put down, but it may also cause "CNS [central nervous system] disorder, obesity, disruptions in adipose tissue physiology, hepatic damage, CRS [Chinese restaurant syndrome] and reproductive malfunctions."[89] Arguably, in small amounts, MSG might be considered harmless, as the human body does have some ability to deal with toxins and chemicals. However, because it makes everything it touches more delicious, it increases our desire to gorge on foods that contain it. Thus, we find ourselves regularly overeating, especially when it comes to unhealthy food stuff, which I feel unable to call food because it is man-made, not God-made.

This, of course, is a double whammy. Not only are we feeding our bodies toxins, but the toxins are causing us to overfill to the point of serious health risk. In a scenario where even a little is a lot, a lot is certainly too much!

Is it All About Moderation?

"Avoid filling the stomach with food and drink.
Overeating exhausts the body and causes illnesses. Follow a
middle way in eating and drinking as this improves the body."
– The Prophet, Muhammad (PBUH)

There are ample classical Islamic sources that discuss the subject of food. In surah Al-Baqarah of the Qur'an, it is stated that we must "eat and drink but not to excess" and that we should "not cast [ourselves] to destruction by [our] own hands" (2:32; 2:195). Although the latter of these teachings may hold meaning unrelated to food, we see both passages as warnings from Allah that seek to prevent us from transgressing the limits that are set to protect us. For when we do, we only harm ourselves. In many examples in the Hadith, we see that it is the middle path that we should adopt, meaning that we should be moderate in our affairs. This includes our relationship with foods.

The concept of moderation is not exclusive to Islam. Time and time again, we see fitness gurus and weight-loss guides telling us that "everything in moderation" is key. Inevitably, you will be exposed to foods that may not be beneficial to your health, so the consumption of beneficial foods should outweigh that of the unbeneficial. I believe most of us have it the other way around.

People often ask me, "Is it okay that I have fast food once a week?" Or, "Can I have a packaged chocolate on cheat day?" However, I am of the strong opinion that there is no moderation when it comes to junk food. As mentioned in the previous chapter, we can feed ourselves and our children whatever we want, but we are not immune to the consequences of our actions. God has given us free will and responsibility, which are the very concepts that separate us from other mammals.

Additionally, there is no moderation when it comes to a chemically laced chocolate bar. A bite or a block – it is all bad for you. Whether it is the preservative that has not been tested or the colour that was unethically taken from insects, it is harmful to your being. Poison is poison, whether you take a gram or a kilogram at a time. The only difference is when the consequences will show up, and this is relative to every other aspect of you. Your diet, environment, genes, liver function, chemical insults your body needs to override every day, quality of sleep, and even your thought processes all determine when symptoms or illness will appear.

In saying this, I am not going to pretend that everyone is perfect all the time – I certainly am not! It really comes down to what moderation means *for you*. For some, moderation might mean having dessert only on the weekend. For others, it might mean abstaining altogether. It is up to you to decide what you are comfortable putting into your body. From an Islamic perspective, it is also dependent on our religious philosophy: the religious calibre set by the Qur'an and prophetic teaching. It is also largely influenced by where you are in your practice of Islam. We are all at different parts of this journey, and my D, E, and F may be your A, B, and C. What is important is to ensure that we are learning and then applying that learning to our lives each and every day, rather than collecting information like a donkey with books tied on its back, as Abdurrahman Dilipak, a renowned researcher and Muslim activist, puts it.

Quality Food and Accountability

When we take ownership of our health, we become better equipped to make decisions that benefit our bodies long-term. Very rarely do we know what we are eating. Therefore, we must be empowered with the knowledge to turn over a food packet and understand exactly what is in it. Quite frankly, if you cannot make sense of the ingredients, it is safe to say you should put that package right back down.

It is undeniable that what we eat has a direct impact on our health, and, relatively speaking, we know very little about it. Sure, we understand that eating too many calories will make us fat and too much soda may rot our teeth, but we rarely turn our minds to the underlying impact that food has on our health and spiritual alignment with God and all His creations. We think food simply enters from one hole and exits from the other, and it certainly does that, but this is only part of the whole truth that we must see. During this journey, which genes are switched on or off, which chemicals and toxins accumulate, and which nutritional deficiencies create illness and symptoms are all determined by the quality of food we eat.

We place a lot of trust in governments, the media, and our favourite social media influencers to tell us what we should – and should not – do to benefit our health. It is true that mass media has a fundamental role to play in the dissemination of information and education about health. It has an enormous influence over society's perceptions and opinions. But because corporate media only distributes content that is newsworthy, it often omits less flashy information. Accordingly, important health data, particularly regarding dietary research and advice, is often under-reported. Remember, too, that these companies have lobbyists in every avenue: science and research, marketing, ethics. No wonder it is hard for us to stay afloat in this sea of information that is naturally biased towards whatever brings in more profit.

It is a challenge knowing that corporate media does not speak much on the importance of food and its impact on our health. I am not saying that I have not seen my share of news headlines stating that "food X" gives you cancer, only to be substituted for "food Y" the following fortnight.

We each need to actively learn about what we consume and why we consume it. For example, what *exactly* is in that frozen meal you defrost every Wednesday night for dinner? Do you know what all those little numbers and ingredients mean on the back of the box? If the answer is no, then it is your responsibility to educate yourself. No one else is going to do it for you, and, quite frankly, no one genuinely cares about your health more than you. It is your responsibility to do the work of demystifying. Yes, it is a challenge, and it takes time and energy, but we are lucky to live at a time of endless resources and opportunities. We have places and people to seek health advice from, and then we can make informed and conscious decisions for ourselves. The consciousness that differentiates us from any other mammal is where our responsibility comes from. The Qur'an states that humans – not only Muslims – are the vicegerents of

Allah on the Earth, and we can choose to live life in the spiritual void, which is an easier task than to take on the responsibility of living life consciously in every facet of it.

Once you start learning exactly what it is that you are eating, you will automatically find yourself making better food choices. After all, no one intentionally wants to fill their bodies with toxic chemicals. Unless, of course, there is subconscious sabotage associated with trauma and a lack of self-worth, which we discussed in previous chapters. In that case, clearly, mental health work must be done to remove the fog.

The ground rule when deciding what to eat always boils down to common sense and what is in sync with nature and aligned with our spiritual ethos. For example, learning which fruits and vegetables are naturally grown in which seasons would be a great place to start in terms of nutrition requirements for your body in alignment with the seasons.

We can also reduce our exposure to packaged foods as much as possible. Instead of consuming tinned chickpeas, we can take the effort to soak some chickpeas the night before or boil them for a little longer to use in soups and salads. This is better than using the salt-laced version that has been leaching plastics and heavy metals from the can because it has been sitting on a shelf for three years. The concept of canned food is genius, but it was not designed for you and me originally. It was designed by the French government in the late 18th century to preserve food for their army and navy.

The Prophet's Example

When we look at Islam as a whole, there is not only much about what to eat but also *why* we eat certain foods. Of course, not everything can fit in the Qur'an. If it could, the Qur'an would be hundreds of volumes large.

Instead, it covers everything important in general light, and whatever needs further emphasis is included in the life of the Prophet (PBUH) and his narrations. His recommendations support current medical studies in the areas of preventative medicine, herbal medicine, nutrition, and the treatment of ailments.

Prophet Muhammad (PBUH) would only consume two meals a day, and our goal, perhaps, is to get as close to his lifestyle as possible, as this is in attunement with the needs of our physical and spiritual bodies. Generally, one of those meals was light, for example, dates or a barley dish for breakfast. There is an authentic saying on the importance of not skipping breakfast and another I will mention here on not skipping dinner: "Do not leave dinner even if it is only a handful of days because abandoning it makes one weak."[90]

The dangers of obesity and overeating are sufficiently highlighted in the Prophet's words: "What I fear most about my community are developing a belly, oversleeping and idling."[91] This truth has come to fruition for more than 39 million children, 340 million adolescents, and 650 million adults who are regarded as obese.[92] In a world where Muslims are the highest population, it is a sad sight to see that 75 percent of the world's population is 'overfat'.[93]

I actually could not find any information on whether the Prophet (PBUH) ate lunch, and almost all sources say that he ate twice a day, with very few suggesting he ate once a day. This goes against the current narrative of three meals and two snacks a day, which is, in essence, actually quite harmful, as the body is constantly expending energy digesting and breaking down food and, thus, not leaving very much for anything else.

There is a plethora of evidence that speaks of the benefits of fasting that we will explore together in the upcoming chapters, and this was indeed His way of life. Needless to say, eating less reduces the risk of obesity and reduces cholesterol levels, two very favourable outcomes.

"The Prophet's main requirement of food was that it should be lawful and clean, as well as beneficial for the body. His two meals consisted of breakfast and dinner, as is recommended by modern medicine. In a nutshell, the amount of intake and eating etiquette recommended by our Prophet is allocating 'one third of the stomach for food, one-third for drink, and one-third for air'."[94]

As a spirit in a physical vessel – or a physical vessel that contains a spirit – we cannot just look at food as something that satiates the physical body the same way we cannot look at the spirit and work on only the spiritual body. We must address both, in moderation, as Islam is the moderate path. The physical body is left to return back to the soil, while the spiritual migrates to a fourth dimension, no longer requiring a physical vessel. Our goal is to get there through conscious living.

CHAPTER SIX

THE JURISPRUDENCE OF FOOD FROM AN ISLAMIC PERSPECTIVE

For some of us who practice Islam, little inward work is done, for the vast majority, actually. Instead, we exert most of our energy in the external work: wearing the hijab (head covering), the act of physical prayer, and attending the mosque. However, there are deeper layers to our spirituality, and I cannot help but to think that, most of the time, the physical actions are void of the spiritual understanding and acknowledgement of *why* certain things are done. Perhaps it is easier to change the outward prior to changing the inward. Turning inward and tuning in, aligning, digesting, assimilating, understanding, and healing is a lot harder than just making the physical changes.

Food and Spirituality

The modern Muslim is often surprised when they are shown the direct correlation between their food and their religion. Though many Muslims are aware that the classical Islamic texts make reference to food, most do not take it further by analysing *how* or *why* what goes into the body affects spirituality.

Islam teaches that what goes into the body impacts its ability to perform its physical and psychological functions and consciously connect to its creator. In layman's terms, what you eat affects your relationship with Allah. If this is your first time hearing this, it might sound a little abstract – but hear me out.

The concept of health and wellness is a core philosophy of our religion. It is in the Qur'an and conveyed via the practices of our prophet, Muhammad (PBUH). The body is just a physical vessel in which we manifest our spiritual selves; hence, its wellness determines the wellness of our spiritual and emotional selves.

Self-care is not just about getting a massage after a long week or having a coffee with friends. The true essence of self-care lies within the foundations of self-compassion and respect for our physical and emotional bodies, which perform their jobs on the physical earth plane. Thus, lack of self-care is when the spiritual body is void, even when the physical body is not. However, I believe things that are obligatory to the Muslim, such as our five daily prayers, when practiced, are actually self-care in and of themselves.

This concept of self-care includes what we eat, what we drink, and how food gets to our plates. Ethical farming practices, treating animals with dignity, and whether vegetables are sprayed with poisons are all important factors. We also need to consider the people working in the farms and factories that produce and supply our food: whether they are treated well, paid well, and have – at minimum – their basic human needs met.

As you read this, you may be thinking, *Are you serious? Considering all of these things is hard work.* Of course it is! Everything worth doing takes time, love, and patience. We are only responsible for what we have conscious awareness of, but we are also responsible for learning what we do not know – and free will makes us accountable to learn from cradle to grave.

When a client who frequently eats fast food fish burgers walks through my virtual doors, I take them to the next level. I introduce them to tinned tuna, jarred tuna, and then wild caught fish until we are at a place where we question the ethics of fishing altogether. Then we decide whether the benefit of, for example, obtaining the omega-3 through the fish outweighs the periodic disadvantages that it causes to the human body, to the earth plane, and to the fish itself. However, no individual starts at the same place on the journey to better holistic health. Someone may be in the middle chapter of their journey, and another may be at the beginning, while another is closer to the finish line. As practitioners, it is our job to meet people where they are and hold their hands and continue to guide them throughout the journey, free of judgement and conscious of their abilities within their intellectual, social, economic, political, spiritual, and religious means.

If someone is consuming fish burgers through a fast-food chain, I need to be gentle with them. I cannot say, "My goodness, you shouldn't eat fish at all because of mercury and plastics, and we have massive holes in our seas due to overfishing." This is far more than they can tolerate in one bite. It is important to take everything in this book one bite at a time. Believe me, I went through my teenage years eating fast food, cornflakes in cow's milk with a tablespoon of processed white sugar, and spoonful after spoonful of Nutella from its plastic jar. Much like any typical teenager, I had no conscious awareness of anything other than the impact of the calories on my physical body. I observed the elephant solely from a linear plane, the only consideration being my physical appearance.

I share this with you in immense vulnerability so while you read this book, you do not imagine me to be on a pedestal, someone who makes no mistakes in health and nutrition and, instead, acknowledge that I am one of you, sharing my own mistakes and experiences, one page at a time. I want you to hold your hand on your heart and tell yourself it is okay for you to pick this book up and feel safe, no matter where you are on your journey of conscious living, and be okay to continue, whether you do that through crawling, walking, or running.

The struggle is real. Every single day I battle with my ego. Some days I win, and some days I do not. Having knowledge and conscious awareness does not mean that we will not repeat the same mistakes or that every single day we are conscious. Our consciousness, ego, and self-righteousness swing like a pendulum, and this is okay. God created us as humans, with egos attached to our physical and spiritual bodies. We are not as angels, who only fulfill God's commandments, but as beings of light and darkness, as beings who are fully able to become light, as beings whose own darkness weakens their spiritual bodies but strengthens their physical bodies. This is why repentance is so important for Muslims. There is a whole chapter in the Qur'an called 'repentance' (surah At-Tawbah) that starts with, "O My servants who have committed excesses against their own souls, do not despair of the mercy of Allah. Indeed, Allah will forgive all sins. Indeed, He is the All-forgiving, the All-merciful."

Isn't that interesting, "… who have committed excess against their own souls"? Isn't it interesting that as creatures with free will, the holy book handballs the responsibility to us? Everything that happens to you that is good comes from Allah, and everything that does not is your own hands' doing. Ouch! That hurts, doesn't it? It sure shook me when I first read that verse, correctly translated as, "Whatever reaches to you of good, is from Allah, but whatever befalls you of evil, is from yourself" (Qur'an 4:79).

Eating ethically means that we must also consider whether chemicals, packaging, or processing has affected or interfered with the flow of the food's divine energy. Will the food serve me by connecting me to the divine? Will it provide me with the mental and physical power to serve my lord in this physical vessel? Or will it draw me away from him?

How Intention Shapes Our Reality

In the late 90s and early 2000s, Masaru Emoto shook the world with his research on water. I read about Dr Emoto's work through his book, *The Hidden Messages in Water*.[95] Dr Emoto was a Japanese scientist, who did extensive research on how water responds to emotional language. So, in essence, what he did was label multiple jars that contained distilled water with words that were positively associated, such as beauty, passion, and happiness, while others were labelled with negatively associated words, such as hate, disgust, and evil.

The water was observed under a microscope after it was frozen, and Dr Emoto found that the positively associated jars had formed crystals that were symmetrical and beautiful, and the negatively associated crystals were fragmented and all over the place in terms of their patterns.

I actually did this very experiment myself out of curiosity; except I added rice. I had one jar with words of affirmation, one with negativity, and another I just abandoned. In as short as two weeks, the abandoned and insulted jars of water and rice had become black, and the water was brown. However, the jar with positive affirmations was as perfect as it was on day one. All of the jars were in the same room.

Of course, Dr Emoto's work was mostly criticised and looked down on, as things are when we cannot understand them or when they surpass our five senses. However, in reality, his work showed us the importance of thoughts and how thoughts affect the physical realm. This is true about the human brain and the human mind, which affect our physical bodies.

Eating Consciously

We start eating with bismillah (in the name of Allah) to bring awareness to the fact that the food was provided by Him and that He is the giver, the sustainer, and the taker of life. We sit and eat with consciousness rather than just to satiate our palates.

Let us look at this from the perspective that the Qur'an is a cure for all but death. You may think, *How can words cure me of an ailment? I've read them all, and I'm still sick.* However, the science behind it is very clear now.

In quantum physics, we acknowledge that everything is constantly in motion, continuously moving and changing. When somebody recites the Qur'an, the very vibration of the voice does two things. Firstly, it activates the vagus nerve, which then activates the parasympathetic nervous system, placing the body in a state of calm, healing, and repair.[96] When activating this process, correct pronunciation is important. Secondly, when the words are felt or heard by our cells, the cells start to oscillate and vibrate in a manner that allows them to detoxify by releasing exosomes. The release of exosomes means the cell is cleansing, and a clean cell is a healthy cell.

Therein lies the answer to how the recitation of certain words, pronounced in a certain way, can affect the way our cells function. This is why music can either be very harmful to the physical and spiritual body or, depending on the instruments used, very healing.

There are numerous references to the importance of healthy eating in the Qur'an, some of which we explored in the previous chapter. To be truly healthy in Islam, a person must be physically and spiritually conscious and live in accordance with the way of life prescribed by Allah, which does not disconnect the physical from the spiritual. We already explored the Hadith, 'one third of your stomach', that inspired the title of this book. As discussed, food, water, and empty space are all given equal weight. None is more important than the other; they each work together to unite spiritual and physical wellness.

Think about it like this. What we eat affects our energy levels, emotions, sleep quality, and fitness. If we eat too much, we feel lethargic and tired. If we eat too little, we become weak and fatigued. Making the right food choices can be the difference between fractured sleep and a good night's rest, which will either leave us feeling irritated and unfocused or productive and composed the following day. Our level of composure further affects our relationships with our partners, our children, and our extended communities. It can also influence how consciously we behave and how present we are. All of this affects a Muslim's relationship with Allah.

When we are low on energy, we lack the fortitude to do the good things that are required of us. Even if we plan to complete a beneficial deed, we may give up because it is too much effort. We begin to slip up and make poor choices, as we do not have the strength to abstain from our "lusts and desires."[97] And this is just the physical truth, not the spiritual truth.

What about the fact that prayer is not as healing or transformative as we intend it to be? When we eat too much, we become weighed down, both physically and mentally. We grow in size, which physically limits our ability to perform prayer and attend the mosque. Mental and physical fatigue leave us unable to truly observe our creator. Our mental state is prone to negativity when we are not feeling our physical best – a direct consequence of poor diet – which makes us act in negative ways, including having negative thoughts about the Lord.[98] Thus, keeping a clear and positive mind is essential to preserving spirituality. As Hasan Al Basri once said: "The believer assumes the best about his Lord, so he does the best deeds. The sinner assumes the worst about his Lord, so he does evil deeds."

Islamic food consumption is logical and rather straightforward. You do not need to be a Muslim to be a conscious consumer, and not every conscious consumer is Muslim. Simple logical connections with our earth, such as eating in season, preventing overconsumption, exercising regularly, and waiting for a meal to digest before consuming another, can help us all live healthier lives. If you are Muslim, it is your duty to try to live in accordance with the basic core fundamentals of the 1,400-year-old food and lifestyle philosophy gifted to us by the Qur'an and Muhammad (PBUH).

Halal Food

"Allah has forbidden you dead meat, and blood, and the flesh of swine, and that which any other name has been invoked besides that of Allah. But if one is forced by necessity, without wilful disobedience, nor transgressing due limits, then he is guiltless. For Allah is oft – forgiving Most Merciful."
– Qur'an 2:173

Eating halal is one of the most recognisable practices of a Muslim, and, as time goes on, halal certified foods are becoming more accessible in supermarkets and restaurants across the Western World. I often see products in Coles and Woolworths branded with the big halal tick. On the face of it, this is, of course, positive. However, with Australia's laws surrounding the slaughter and sale of meat for consumption, one has to wonder: is halal meat in Australia really worthy of its accreditation?

Halal means permissible under Islamic (or Sharia) law. It is a universal term that can refer to anything that is in alignment with the light of Islamic jurisprudence. For example, food, drink, meat, pharmaceuticals, and cosmetics can all be halal or not.

When we talk about halal meat, we are talking about meat that is free of anything that is prohibited under Islamic law – for example, pig or carnivorous animal meat and by-products – and has been prepared in accordance with our law.

Under Sharia, for meat to be considered halal, it must satisfy the following criteria:

- The animal must be treated well prior to being killed, meaning that it is given the right to sexually reproduce, eat its own foods, and receive ample sunlight, space, love, and compassion.
- The animal must be slaughtered by a sane adult Muslim.
- During slaughter, the name of God must be invoked to stress the sanctity of life and that the animal is being killed for food with the consent of God. Mostly, we acknowledge spiritually that the animal will surrender itself to the slaughterer if the slaughtering is done in the correct way because it knows that, in part, it was created to serve the food chain of the human. In essence, being eaten elevates its status from animal to a part of the protein structure and the genetic material of man, who was created 'above' it.
- The cut must be made at the carotid artery to ensure that the animal is killed immediately and does not experience any additional suffering.
- The knife must be sharp enough to slaughter the animal in one go. To avoid evoking fear, the knife cannot be shown or sharpened in front of the animal. Fear, of course, fills the blood with stress hormones like cortisol, which then end up in the animal flesh that we consume.
- All blood must be allowed to bleed out and completely drain. There are many reasons for this. Looking at it from a health perspective, this gets rid of any pathogens that may have been

lingering in the blood and also decreases exposure to sex and stress hormones from the animal.

As long as meat is prepared this way and does not contain any unlawful products, it is permitted for Muslim consumption.

The challenge with eating halal in Australia is that, by law, all animals must be stunned (rendered unconscious) before they are hand slaughtered or slaughtered on machines. Stunning occurs either by electrified water bath or gas. For example, chickens have to be removed from their crates and shackled for the electrical stunning process. For gas stunning, birds either remain in their crates or are transferred to a conveyor system that takes them through the gas. Once unconscious, the birds' throats are cut, allowing them to bleed out and die.[99]

Stunning poses a threat to meat being permissible under Islamic law, even if the animal has otherwise been cut according to halal standards. During the stunning process, it is possible for the animal to die, and the Qur'an prohibits consuming the meat of an animal that has not been slaughtered according to Islamic law. If an animal dies during stunning and is cut later, at face value, it defies chapter two verse 173 of the Qur'an: "He has only forbidden you what dies of itself, and blood, and flesh of swine, and that over which any other (name) than (that of) Allah has been invoked; but whoever is driven to necessity, not desiring, nor exceeding the limit, no sin shall be upon him; surely Allah is Forgiving, Merciful."

The other challenge is the stress animals go through during the stunning process, as meat cannot be halal if the animal has experienced suffering. Food affects our spiritual and physical wellbeing. Sometimes I say, "If you eat a headless chook, you will feel like one." If an animal is not slaughtered compassionately and in accordance with Islamic principles, it will pass on its suffering through its meat. When an animal feels distress from knowing that it is going to die, due to seeing blood from an animal cut prior, hearing another animal's cries, or simply by understanding what is happening as it runs through the factory farm conveyor belt, it is building levels of adrenaline and cortisol within its bloodstream. By consuming this meat, you will increase your own levels of these stress hormones, which can linger in your blood and affect your mental and emotional wellbeing.[100]

When it comes to stunning, there is some debate around what is considered ethical, with groups like the RSPCA implying that it is more humane than slaughtering animals while they are lucid.[101] However, let us put all this aside and acknowledge that we just mentioned a verse in surah Al-Baqarah that confirmed that an animal that is dead before it is slaughtered cannot be consumed as halal meat. We know that, much of the time, animals that are stunned prior to hand slaughtering have already died. This was made evident in a paper released by the Australian National Imams Council, which stated that controlled atmospheric stunning (CAS) was not permissible. However, it is the main method used by the largest abattoirs in Australia. And I quote: "Upon careful assessment and consideration of the report results, the absence of VITAL signs and ECG indication, the Australian Fatwa Council has concluded that the practice of CAS stunning, in its **current** form, is **NOT** fit for halal consumption under the Islamic laws and principles of halal slaughter."[102]

Now, I want to make it clear that I am *not* advocating for animal suffering. In fact, I support living on a plant-based diet the majority of the time, with very minimal exposure to meat. We should live as close as possible to Islamic standards, which have been violated and adulterated by our culture.

Kindness for the Creatures of God

When Muhammad (PBUH) disseminated the Qur'an, the practice of slaughtering animals was not put through the lens of an industrialised society like today's. While the current meat and dairy market is filled with large-scale abattoirs and artificial insemination practices, in the past people hand raised and slaughtered animals themselves, with the time and space to honour them properly. These days, cows, chickens, sheep, and goats are massacred by the thousands. In this holocaust, there is no process for honouring the animal. Everything is done mechanically, taking the fact that the animal has a life and a right over us out of the equation.

The Qur'an describes "the slaves of God" as being "those who walk on the Earth in humility" (25:63). Scholars have interpreted this verse and others like it to mean that Muslims are to protect nature's many bounties given to them by the Almighty. I beg to understand: which part of our relationship with animals is humble? Many may argue that, given the current population of the world, factory farming is the only way to go. I would stand strong in my stance that if we ate like Muhammad (PBUH), thus did not consume meat or dairy daily, there would be no need for profit-driven abattoirs that exploit animals on a physical and spiritual level.

When the human (not the Muslim) was stated to be a vicegerent for all of creation, I am certain that God based this decision on our free will, consciousness, and ability to discern right from wrong. He wanted us to put our intellect to good use and protect our environment and the living beings that inhabit it. Instead, we use our smarts to exploit animals and drive a profit-based industry to the trillions.

In Islam, humans are required to be compassionate toward all animals: "Whoever is kind to the creatures of God, is kind to himself."[103] It is not whoever is kind to a *human*, but whoever is kind to a *creature*.

In fact, there is a story of a Sahaba (companion of the Prophet) who would leave crumbs on an ant hill. When his friend asked him why he would bother feeding crumbs to ants, his response was, "I fear that they will testify against me on the day of judgement." There is a level of consciousness that perhaps you could argue is not necessarily reachable for us these days. However, our job is to at least try. Our Islamic obligation to act with morality is second to none, and we must uphold these standards in our lives to the best of our ability.

Islam prohibits acts like selling animals and pets. Why? Because while we are obliged to protect and preserve them and their natural habitat, we do not own them. Unlike animals, we have the ability to make a choice. Most animals mainly eat out of need, but humans eat for pleasure. We eat when we are sad, angry, happy, bored, or dissociated. We turn to food to fill a spiritual void. The animal does not have the free will to make decisions beyond its need to survive. It generally kills what it needs to eat, and it only eats to its fill.

What Is the Alternative to Eating Meat?

If we are to eat meat in this industrialised landscape, then perhaps stunning an animal prior to slaughter *is* more humane than the alternative, which is hundreds of animals witnessing one another have their throats slit in a gas chamber. Perhaps, when dealing with such a large quantity of meat, there really is no better alternative than the pre-stunning process. However, if the essence of the Qur'an is to limit the suffering of an animal before slaughter, how can we justify today's meat manufacturing practices that mistreat animals and violate their rights? Even the most 'ethical' abattoirs are horrifying scenes of pain and torture. Maybe, the answer is that we cannot justify this practice. Perhaps, to truly eat halal, we must stop eating commercially produced meat altogether.

It is at this juncture that we must ask ourselves: why do we eat so much meat, anyway? I suppose, just like most other people across the globe, we were told that it was beneficial for our health, a story inherited from our mothers and grandmothers. So, without question, we have continued to implement a carnivorous diet. But, eventually, enough of us will develop the health problems associated with the consumption of meat and dairy and realise that something does not add up.

As Omar RA warns us, it may be very challenging to turn back from the addiction. In the Muwatta, Omar RA, who was a dear friend of the Prophet (PBUH) and became the second caliphate of Islam upon Muhammad's passing, says, "Beware of meat for in meat there is an addiction as there is in wine." What level of wisdom did these men have to know that certain areas of the brain light up when we consume meat and dairy? Dairy, specifically, gives us the same pleasure as a stimulant drug. For example, cheese may be "addictive in a way similar to drugs because of a chemical called casein, which is found in dairy products and can trigger the brain's opioid receptors."[104]

Perhaps 1,400 years ago, there was no science to back up many of the claims around food, and some may have seemed exaggerated or unnecessary. However, we now understand that many of the claims aimed to inspire current and future generations to make favourable food choices.

I have *never* heard of anyone being hospitalised for protein deficiency, except in Third World countries. However, extreme starvation can cause deficiencies in almost everything, not just protein. I do know that cardiovascular disease – an epidemic driven by diets that contain too much meat, dairy, and refined foods, including sugars and salts – is responsible for 118 deaths per day in Australia.[105] That is a lot of people losing their lives to preventable diseases. This is the real epidemic.

A Plant-Based Diet for the Conscious Human

Of course, I am a realist. I understand that asking families to give up eating meat entirely is a *big* ask. Besides, for a lot of Muslims, the halal certification is enough to deem consumption permissible.

Trying to live in accordance with the Qur'an means making conscious choices about what we do and how we act. Even if we accept that meat in Australia satisfies the requirements of halal, at the very least, we must be conscious of where and whom it comes from and how it is produced. Whenever we purchase or consume meat, we must ask ourselves whether we are making the most ethical choice. We do this by turning our minds to whether it is organic, sustainably farmed (as much as possible), and grass-fed. Before we eat meat, we must always consider whether doing so is necessary. There are truly no pitfalls when we reduce consumption or omit it from our diets, as long as we meet our nutritional needs with other foods.

The jihad – the struggle of the soul – is real. Every single day we are obliged by social, intellectual, and financial standards to do what is right. It is not a simple or linear journey, but it is one that is placed upon every single sane Muslim. Our job is to strive. We must consider the journey, not the destination. It does not matter so much whether we complete it, as intention and application hold the most weight. Our job is to set goals and move forward each and every day with as clear a conscience as possible because once we are consumed by shame, it becomes even easier to mask this emotion with food and even harder to disconnect from it.

Tayyib Food

"For he [the Prophet Muhammad (PBUH)] commands them what is just and forbids them what is evil; he allows them as lawful what is good and pure and prohibits them what is bad and impure."
– Qur'an 7:157

When we see the word halal, tayyib will not be far away. Although there is no direct English translation, tayyib means wholesome, pure, organic, and clean. Food must meet tayyib requirements under Islamic law. Therefore, if food is not tayyib, it cannot be halal and is not permissible for the Muslim to consume.

For example, if we are to use the term tayyib in relation to beef, *as well as* looking at whether it is halal, we would need to consider things like:

- Was the cow raised happily?
- Was it given sunlight and its natural feed?
- Was it allowed to naturally reproduce and achieve sexual satiation?
- Was it given love, compassion, and friends?
- Like humans, animals are social beings who get depressed when left alone. Was it kept in an environment that was clean and conducive to its positive mental and physical health?
- As much as possible, was the animal treated fairly and given all its rights?

When we look at the Australian law around halal, it does not consider any level of tayyib. So, is it truly permissible for us to consume commercial halal meats? Or is it time to raise our voices, as this form of food affects us in ways that are immeasurably damaging to the physical and spiritual body?

Like halal, tayyib is not just used in reference to meat. For example, if we were talking about wheat, we would ask:

✧ From where were the seeds obtained?

✧ How were they managed?

✧ Who harvested the wheat?

✧ Were the workers given their rights in terms of healthy, ethical working conditions and reasonable pay?

✧ Is the wheat the result of genetic modification?

✧ Was its gene pool changed for man's benefit or financial profit?

✧ Was it hybridised, and does this process contribute to more cons than pros?

✧ Was the water used in its production clean and pure?

✧ Did it grow in its natural state or in an artificial state, for example, using artificial lighting and growing in water only?

The answers to these questions determine whether or not a product is tayyib. To be conscious consumers, we must vigorously dissect the origin of our food, as it impacts both our spiritual and physical vessels and also our environment and global pollution footprint. Is halal certified food that lacks the concept of tayyib equal to organic food that lacks halal certification? I do not know. However, I implore you to ask these questions in relation to Islamic jurisprudence, to ponder the questions that are rarely asked. No answers are ever obtained without dissecting information and applying it intellectually to the question. Your intellect was not given to you for nothing. It was provided to help you ascertain right from wrong and good from bad.

Organic Food

We can make a broad assumption and state that organic can equate to tayyib, but, in reality, legislation around the world varies regarding what does and does not meet this classification. In Australia, it is important to understand the difference between 'organic' and 'certified organic' foods. Foods that are advertised as simply being organic do not actually have any accreditation or formal checks to ensure the produce meets organic standards. In essence, this means that a manufacturer can claim that its product is organic without it being true. However, making a "misleading, false or deceptive claim" about the organic status of a product is illegal in Australia.[106]

In contrast, certified organic products have passed a number of checks performed by a regulatory body. Generally, for a product to meet certified organic requirements, it must be "free from human-made fertilisers, pesticides, growth regulators, and GMOs."[107] There is no mandatory certification requirement for organic produce. Instead, various private certification companies can grant this label for a fee, which means that some companies simply do not label their produce organic because they do not want to pay for certification.[108]

Similarly, there is no established organic standards body for domestic products. However, organic standards for exports and imports are regulated by the *Trade Practices Act 1974* (Cth), the National Standard for Organic and Bio-Dynamic Produce, and Organic and Biodynamic Products – AS6000:2015, though the latter is voluntary. Penalties are imposed on companies who purport their produce to be organic when it is not.[109]

So, when we consider whether our food is tayyib, we must look to where it comes from and how it is produced. If our food *is* labelled organic, it is important to understand what that actually means and whether it meets the Islamic standards of tayyib.

Factory Farming

In Australia and many other countries around the world, for the most part, meat and dairy is factory farmed. Animals are fed and raised to produce meat and dairy. This is not a natural process, but it is hugely profitable.

Let us take cows, for example. I once attended an abattoir and farm that manufactured milk, and I watched how semen was artificially collected from bulls. During the process, the bull is shown a cow but is not necessarily allowed to touch it. Just as the male human becomes sexually aroused by visual stimuli, the sight of the cow gets the bull ready to ejaculate into an artificial vagina, which is basically a long rubber tube. The semen is collected, examined under a microscope, and analysed to determine its quality. The ejaculate is then diluted – so the sperm can be used with multiple cows – stored, and frozen. Twenty-four hours later, a portion from each batch is defrosted and tested for quality.[110] The highest quality semen is then used to artificially inseminate the cows.

The size of the offspring matters most: how big they will be and how much meat they will produce. If the offspring is male, it will most likely be sold as a calf, without being raised on its own mother's milk because we need that for our cappuccinos and cheese platters. Thus, the bull becomes a veal. If it is female, it will be continuously impregnated to produce milk until it either becomes too sick or too old. Then it will be slaughtered and sold off as meat. These processes are far from tayyib and far from what the Prophet (PBUH) envisioned when he spoke of proper eating practices.

In the Code of Accepted Farming Practice for the Welfare of Cattle, it states that if any cattle have a tumour pre-slaughter, the abattoir must address it.[111] This, in essence, means that the tumour is cut out, and the meat is still deemed acceptable for public consumption. The rise in human cancer rates is alarming, and this set me off on a journey to see whether it had anything to do with consuming meat that may have been affected by tumours or cancers.

The World Health Organisation already classifies red meat as a Group 2A carcinogen (likely carcinogenic to humans) and processed meats as a Group 1 carcinogen (almost certainly carcinogenic to humans).[112] A carcinogen, by definition, is a "substance, organism or agent capable of causing cancer."[113]

Environmental Considerations

"Eat and drink from the provision of Allah, and do not commit abuse on the earth, spreading corruption."
– Qur'an 2:60

Waste

As vicegerents, our duty is to act as guardians of the earth. We are free to use the environment, but we must never abuse or exploit it. So, for our diet to satisfy both halal and tayyib requirements, we must ensure that we are turning our minds to the environmental impact our food has on the planet. For each product we use or consume, we need to consider the carbon footprint of its packaging, the pollution caused by its transportation, and, especially in the case of animal products, how much food and water it takes to produce.

It is no secret that the meat and dairy industries have enormous impacts on the environment. In fact, studies have shown that it takes 5,000 to 20,000 litres of water to produce just one kilogram of beef, generating 99.48 kilograms of greenhouse gas emissions per kilogram.[114] Additionally, meat and dairy farming have deleterious effects on our native vegetation due to the vast amount of land that has been – and continues to be – cleared for cattle grazing.

As vicegerents on Earth, it is our responsibility to be vigilant against mistreating the planet and the environment. By reducing our consumption of meat and dairy, we can reduce our ecological footprint. Of course, when it comes to living sustainably, we can never be perfect. But as long as we each do our part, we are living in accordance with Islamic principles. Here are some simple actions you can take to reduce your ecological footprint:

- ✧ Bring your own bag from home when grocery shopping
- ✧ Pay more to buy Australian-made products
- ✧ Chose a shampoo bar over a bottle to reduce plastic use
- ✧ Opt for organic dairy to encourage mainstream dairy businesses to be more mindful of farming practices
- ✧ Purchase olives and similar foods in glass jars, which take more energy to produce but can be reused, rather than plastic.

When it comes to reducing our ecological footprints, we should do what we can within our own emotional, physical, mental, and financial abilities. God does not ask for anything outside of this. We are to learn and grow each and every day as we work on creating a better connection with our lord and the world around us through conscious living. There will always be compromise, and doing our best at every possible moment is what matters most.

Just the other day, I was shopping, and I bought a packet of dairy-free, chocolate-coated rice crackers. The same company sold them in mini packs of six in plastic wrap or a larger 200-gram packet, also in plastic wrap. I choose the latter. Why? Because I could always divide the snacks and put them in my own containers when popping it in the kids' lunchboxes. Yes, they were still wrapped in plastic, but it was less than what was used for the mini packets.

To me, this was a win. Now, did my purchase still contribute to global pollution? It sure did – the product used plastic. However, I had made a conscious effort to choose the option that would cost the environment less. Would it have been ideal to not have purchased it at all? Of course! But we all know that level of perfection takes work. We are all works in progress, and we must come from a place of self-compassion as much as possible.

Sometimes, as a busy mum, you run out the door and forget your keep cup or your reusable bags and instead buy a takeaway coffee and grab some plastic bags for the shopping. Let's be real – this happens to the best of us. But it is important to ensure that you come from a place of understanding and compassion towards yourself so you do not lose the motivation to keep steadfast in your commitment to remain the vicegerent that God has decreed you to be in the holy book.

Pesticides and Herbicides

There are huge ethical issues with pesticides that make our foods far from tayyib, ethical, or organic. Food that is sprayed poses huge risks to our health. It is not pseudoscience to say that pesticides, which are widespread in Australia and the USA, not only kill insects but also kill the bacteria that make up the soil's microbiome.[115] We are supposed to get our beneficial bugs and viruses – yes, viruses are also a part of our healthy microbiome – from fruits and vegetables. They are beneficial to our gut flora and promote a healthy digestive system and body overall. Ideally, these beneficial bugs would be transferred from the soil to the plants, then from the plants through to us. Pre-pasteurisation, we would also get some of these bacteria from dairy. Think of cow's milk like human breastmilk – it is full of beneficial bugs that set up the body and immune system.

You may have heard of Agent Orange, which the United States military implemented as part of its chemical warfare program during the Vietnam war. Designed purely for plant use, Agent Orange was a herbicide that was mixed up to 20 times its strength to deforest wide areas of vegetation in Vietnam to expose opposition forces. Due to its harsh chemical composition, which created large amounts of 2,3,7,8-tetrachlorodibenzo-p-dioxin (TCDD), a type of dioxin, Agent Orange had widespread and devastating effects on both the Vietnamese and veteran communities. Millions of cases of cancer, auto immunity, and birth defects began emerging in the wake of its use. Because dioxin can remain present in soil for years, complications from Agent Orange continue to arise today, many decades later.[116]

Though the spraying of Agent Orange (dioxin) has largely been discontinued – there are some unverified reports of it being used today – other harmful pesticides remain prevalent. Since 1996, the use of Roundup – a pesticide containing glyphosate, a known carcinogenic – on crops has increased significantly. Although banned in many European countries due to worrying evidence regarding its effects on human health, Roundup continues to be used in Australia. The dumping of this pesticide has created huge residues in our water supply and impacted the quality of the water and food used to sustain livestock.[117]

Roundup has also been shown to lead to serious long-term health issues, particularly cancer. In 2018, US man Dewayne Johnson successfully sued Roundup's manufacturer, Bayer (previously known as Monsanto, the company who also produced Agent Orange), for $289 million. Johnson developed non-Hodgkin's lymphoma from using the product over a sustained period in his job as a groundskeeper, prompting the lawsuit and demand for compensation.[118]

Looking at the overuse of pesticides from a different perspective, we see that some bugs, such as Lactobacillus and Bifidobacterium, and some enterococcus species can become resistant to spraying. This occurs when, due to overexposure, a bug develops an innate ability to survive chemicals that once would have killed it.[119] The bugs that are resistant to the pesticide reproduce, creating a pest that is now unmanageable using the original chemical. When this happens, we need to find a stronger form of intervention to combat the bugs. In fact, sometimes, we develop genetically modified seeds that can withstand the effects of the pesticide or herbicide. In essence, we are trying to find solutions to problems that we create ourselves: man-made cures for man-made illnesses.

Although overuse of pesticides can increase bacteria resistance, the converse is also true. Due to the microbial imbalances, possibly caused by excessive chemical use, bacterial strains are becoming extinct. In the case of some of these strains, we have not even had the chance to identify their benefits on the human and ecological microbiomes. This is a huge loss. There are definitely better ways to deal with the management of 'pests' on crops, which the Sufi would probably view as the haq: the right of the insect/animal eating it!

So, tell me then, is the benefit of spraying a crop with cancer-causing, gene-altering chemicals to reduce potential exposure to insects and weeds a fair trade-off? Is it a fair trade-off Islamically, consciously, and ethically? There is a link between pesticides and cancer.[120] Therefore, is it so easy to label a conventional crop that is laced in these pesticides as being Islamically permissible, even though the large body of evidence suggests harm to the human body?

The other concern is the health of workers on these chemical-laced farms. A 2005 New Zealand study on mortality examined workers exposed to a particular herbicide group – phenoxy herbicides and dioxins – and found that cancer rates increased in exposed production workers.[121] Surely, once we apply a more holistic and compassionate approach to our food chain, we will not only reap the rewards of maintaining our health and reversing many health conditions, but we will also be living in accordance with the requirements that level us up to being the vicegerents of all creations.

Use of the Hands in Islam

As we have seen so far, Islam guides its followers through many aspects of daily life, and the use of the hands is no exception. When it comes to eating, the Prophet (PBUH) has various sayings about correct etiquette surrounding hands, including washing practices, which hand to eat with, and which fingers to use.

Eating with the Right Hand

"Each and every one of you should eat with the right hand, drink with the right hand, take with the right hand, give with the right hand. This is because Satan eats with the left hand, drinks with the left hand, gives with the left hand and takes with the left hand."[122]

In Islam, the right hand is considered 'noble'. It is used for shaking hands, waving, dressing, and, of course, eating. Muslims lead with their right side when entering a mosque and turn to their right after saying prayer. The left side, however, is used for the opposite: undressing, exiting the mosque, and blowing the nose. The left hand is also the appendage used for cleaning up after the bathroom. It is the hand that removes impurities. Energetically speaking, the right hand takes, and the left hand gives.

According to tradition, it is essential that a person only eat and drink using their right hand. However, if they are unable to do so – for example, if the person suffers illness or injury – they are permitted to eat and drink using the left. If a person is left-handed, they will be looked upon favourably if they try to eat with their right hand but, again, will not be punished for not doing so.

The Prophet (PBUH) allocated his hands in this way, so the right hand became preferred within Islam. Looking at this from a practical perspective, the reason for the division is obvious. If the left hand is used to perform a physical cleanse, it would be prudent not to use it when consuming food, just in case it has not been washed thoroughly enough to remove all of the microbes and toxins and prevent the spread of disease, protecting the rights of others.

These days, some Muslims think the act of eating only with the right hand is merely a recommendation, arguing that the climate of the time dictated such measures. When we consider the context – for example, there was no toilet paper or cutlery 1,400 years ago – we can see that such a rule was essential to maintain cleanliness. Because it is mentioned in the Islamic law, at the very least, it is important enough to take into consideration.

Eating with Three Fingers

> *"I saw Messenger of Allah (PBUH) eating with*
> *three fingers and licking them after having finished the food."*
> **– Ka'b bin Malik (may Allah be pleased with him)**

When Muhammad ate, he did so using just three fingers: the thumb, the index finger, and the middle finger. He did this as a display of politeness, for to use the entire hand would imply greed. This does not mean that it is impermissible for a Muslim to eat using other means, such as spoons, which are now commonplace. Rather, if a Muslim is to eat with their hands, they should do so using only those three fingers.

It may come as a surprise that eating with our fingers, as opposed to cutlery, comes with health benefits. While using forks and spoons correlates with faster eating, employing our fingers slows down this process. Not only this, but by using our fingers, we restrict our ability to shove large quantities of food into our mouths at once. By taking smaller, slower bites, we give our bodies more time to digest food, which helps prevent overeating. When we give our bodies the space to acknowledge the food it has been given, we can recognise satiety before overindulging.

Washing of the Hands

"Blessing in food lies in washing the hand before and after eating."
– The Prophet Muhammad (PBUH)

It might seem like common sense, but washing the hands is a fundamental part of adhering to Islamic etiquette. Traditionally, Muslims eat, drink, and wash using their hands, so it is essential that high hygiene standards are maintained.

The oral cavity is one of the most disease-breeding parts of the body. Therefore, washing your hands before a meal will ensure that the food is entering your mouth without excess bacteria, viral particles, or any other pathogen, thereby preventing potential illness. There are billions of strains of bacteria within the mouth. Causing an imbalance here will drive imbalances in the whole gut, potentially leading to bacterial infections of the stomach.

As sharing a meal is a common practice in Islam, washing our hands also prevents others from picking up germs that we could pass on to the food. This basic practice demonstrates the absolute sensitivity and care that Islam has in terms of honouring one another.

Other Sunna That Relate to Food

There are various other practices and sayings of the Prophet (PBUH) that relate to food and form part of the Sharia. I have briefly outlined a few here:

1. EAT WHAT IS DIRECTLY IN FRONT OF YOU

When sharing a meal with others, you can only eat what is directly in front of you. You must not reach out and take food that is before someone else. It is considered bad manners for a person to eat from the middle of a platter, as it may be off-putting to fellow dining companions.

In relation to this, the Prophet (PBUH) said, "O young boy, mention Allah's name, eat with your right hand, and eat from what is directly in front of you," and "The blessing descends in the middle of the food, so eat from the edges and do not eat from the middle."[123] There is an exception when consuming dates; in which case, it is permissible to eat from all parts of the plate.

2. SIT DOWN TO DRINK WATER, AND DRINK IT IN SIPS

When drinking water, you should sit down to drink and never gulp it. According to tradition, the Prophet (PBUH) would pause at three intervals when consuming water, removing his mouth from the container at each break.

3. RINSE THE MOUTH AFTER EATING

It is recommended that you rinse your mouth out after eating or drinking, as the Prophet (PBUH) rinsed his mouth after eating and before praying. Rinsing your mouth and gargling activates your parasympathetic nervous system. By doing this, you promote relaxation and deactivate stress. This also promotes digestion of the food you have just consumed.

There is no need for alcohol or similarly based mouthwashes – water is ample for this. Acidic foods, such as lemons, limes, and oranges, have the potential to erode tooth enamel, so it is best to rinse first and then brush a period after food has been consumed.

4. ACKNOWLEDGE ALLAH

It is Sunna to say the words of praise to Allah before or, if not, after you finish eating: "When any one of you eats, let him mention the name of Allah. If he forgets to mention the name of Allah at the beginning, then let him say '*Bismillaahi awwalahu wa aakhirahu* (In the name of Allah at the beginning and at the end)'."[124] This demonstrates your thanks to Allah for the meal before you, your gratitude to be able to pay for the food, and your acknowledgement of the animal who has given up its life to feed you.

It is easy to ascertain that Islam is not just a religion or a particular set of rules, but a way of life. For whoever delves down the rabbit hole, there is a level of insight into details that otherwise could be missed. Islam does not just tell us what to do; it tells us the why and the how, rendering taking action as simple as possible.

CHAPTER SEVEN

FASTING AND PRAYER

As a Muslim, I find it fascinating that we are often the first to implement the newest health and diet trends, including those that align with our Islamic teachings. Are you familiar with 5:2? If not, let me explain. It is one of the many fasting diets that have quickly become popular, and it involves fasting two days out of the seven-day week. Furthermore, piling research demonstrates the health benefits of this approach. Our prophet recommends that we fast two days of the week, and Islamic teachings recommend that Monday and Thursday be those days.

So, what happens to the body when it is in a state of fasting? Many healing processes take place in the fasted state. It is said that Imam Mawawi said it is desirable that the sick person is not forced to take medicine. Further, it was reported that Allah's Messenger (salallāhu 'alaihi wasallam) said: "Do not force your sick ones to eat and drink for indeed Allah (the Mighty and Majestic) feeds them and gives them drink."[125] This was said 1400 years ago, and now we can acknowledge the science behind it.

When the body is in a state of disease or detox, it needs to conserve most of its energy for healing. If we force-feed the sick, in essence, we apply more stress to the body by giving it one more thing to expend energy on instead of allowing that energy to be used by the immune system. When we do this, instead of healing, the body has to use some energy to break down, digest, and assimilate food, which, in essence, diverts it from its actual task of healing. Basically, if we abstain from food for extended periods of time, we allow the body to heal, as it is no longer engaged in digestive processes, which take up a lot of time and energy. Instead, the body is geared up for cleansing, healing, and detoxing. Therefore, fasting may help heal many modern ailments.

You may ask, "How does the body heal if we're not eating and providing it with food and nutrients?" Organs, such as the liver, always store vitamins and minerals, and these reserves are tapped into when we are in a state of fasting. Therefore, most of us should have ample nutrition for the healing process. From a caloric perspective, any weight lost during sickness as a result of abstaining from food is usually recovered as soon as the body regains balance and health.

At night, melatonin largely contributes to the detoxing, healing, and cleansing that happens when we sleep, as sleep is a state of fasting. Whether we like it or not, for 6–8 hours a day, we abstain from food and give the body a chance to heal. However, this process does not solely rely on forgoing food. When the cleansing and detoxing process is unsuccessful, generally due to poor sleep, many of us wake up feeling like we were hit by a bus.

Several factors can contribute to poor sleep and disrupt the healing process, including:

◇ Lowered serotonin levels, which impede our ability to produce melatonin
◇ Digestive issues
◇ Chronic pain

✧ Chronic systemic inflammation

✧ Bladder issues

✧ Anxiety.

It is empowering to acknowledge that not only did the Prophet (PBUH) suggest fasting two days of the week, as he used to fast on Mondays and Thursdays, but it is further mentioned in the Qur'an: "O ye who believe! prescribed unto you is fasting even as it was prescribed unto those before you, that you may become God-conscious" (2:183).

There are also benefits for fasting in the middle of the month, in alignment with the moon, which is another way Islam reiterates the importance of being in synchronicity with the earth plane. The moon begins as a crescent, then waxes until it is full, then wanes until it is a crescent again. The three middle nights of the lunar month are when the moon is full and circular. Therefore, these are the brightest nights of the month. The brightness of these nights is also one of the reasons why the Prophet (SAW) fasted on these days. It was a way of giving thanks to Allah for lighting the dark nights. This would have been particularly poignant at the time of the Prophet (SAW), when electric lighting had not yet been invented.

Fasting is also one of the pillars of faith, of which we have five. The third describes fasting during the month of Ramadan – a holy month for Muslims – as being a 'requirement' to qualify as a Muslim. To follow the path and lifestyle of Muhammad means to experience life in the healthiest, most spiritually connected way possible. This is one way of empowering the body to heal, thus, preventing the accumulation of toxins and chemicals over time.

Many Benefits of Fasting

When fasting was done 1,400 years ago, as either two days of the week and/or three consecutive days of the month, there were no added chemicals in the air, water, or food. Additionally, food was not hybrid, nor was it GMO, and there was no pollution. Unlike modern man, people were not exposed to high levels of chemicals and toxins, yet they still fasted for the spiritual and physical benefits. Can you imagine, if man 1400 years ago, with no toxicity externally, did this to improve his physical health, how much we could benefit from this in our lives with modern pollution?

If fasting purely remained a voluntary act, would many of us fast two days a week and/or three days a month? The answer is possibly not. As God is the one who created us and has our 'manual', he knew that we would not fast if it was not prescribed for us, if it was not a ritual obligation. Ramadan is a month where all Muslims must fast. There are, of course, exceptions to this. Those who are mentally unwell or otherwise diagnosed with a mental health challenge that prevents them from making conscious decisions on their own, children who have not reached puberty, and women who are going through menses or postpartum bleeding are all exempt. So, to give everyone a fair shot at detoxing, healing, and cleansing, God made fasting obligatory, as he knew many of us would otherwise miss out on its plethora of benefits.

A 2018 study found that mice who fasted lived longer than a control group. Mice either fasted for one day every four, one every three, or one every two, and researchers discovered that mice who fasted the most lived the longest. Not only did the mice live longer, but their quality of life improved. They were less prone to diabetes and cancer, and they mostly died of natural causes.[126]

The animals used in the experiment were genetically engineered dwarf mice, which are designed to not respond to the hormone IGF-1 (insulin-like growth factor 1). As the name implies, IGF-1 promotes the growth of every cell in our bodies and keeps them constantly active. We need adequate levels of this hormone when we are young and growing; however, high levels later in life appear to lead to accelerated ageing and cancer.[127]

Interestingly, fasting reduces IGF-1 – and not just in rodents. Fasting also switches on certain repair genes. When we fill our bodies with food, they are only interested in growing and reproducing. Nature does not have a long-term plan for us, so she does not necessarily invest in us in the long run. Once we have reproduced, we become disposable.

When we fast, initially, the body signals the brain to remind us that we are hungry and urges us to find something to eat. If we continue to resist, the body decides that we are not eating because we are in famine. In the past, this would have been normal because there was not an excessive amount of food available. During a famine, there is no point expending energy on growth or reproduction. Instead, the wisest thing the body can do is spend that energy on repair and keeping us in reasonable shape until we reach a period of feast again.

Taking the foot off the accelerator prompts the body to step in and perform some urgent maintenance and repair. Restricting calories also activates a process called autophagy, which means 'self-eating'. During this process, our bodies break down and recycle old and tired cells, and intermittent fasting is a great way to switch on genes that heal and cleanse the body through the autophagy process.

Fasting also increases the production of a protein called brain-derived neurotrophic factor, which stimulates stem cells to turn into nerve cells in the hippocampus. The hippocampus forms the part of the brain essential for learning and memory. Why would the hippocampus increase stimulation while fasting? From an evolutionary perspective, it makes a lot of sense because when resources are low, people need to be at their smartest and fastest.

Does that not make you ponder the idea that every lifestyle recommendation in Islam is for our benefit? Imagine how many days of our lives we lose due to the accumulation of toxins in our bodies. This may be why humans have gone from living hundreds of years a thousand years ago to us wowing at anyone who lives beyond the age of 90.

Philosophically, fasting reminds Muslims of the less fortunate and reinforces the importance of gratitude. When we fast, we are not only able to sympathise with others who may not have food, but we can empathise because we have experienced genuine moments of intense hunger. We have first-hand experience, which is crucial in obtaining a deeper understanding. So, when you are assessing the benefits of fasting on the physical plane, I acknowledge that there is also a deep and intense blessing and growth of the spiritual and mental planes of the human body.

This brings us to a critically important philosophy about Islam, which is that anything that is suggested to be done benefits both the physical and the spiritual body equally.

The Power of Movement and Prayer

Do you know how we obtain marbled meat? We are certainly not going back to talking about halal and tayyib slaughter; however, this is relevant to the discussion on movement. Wagyu is a form of beef that is obtained from cows, and these cows in particular are cooped up in small sheds and are unable to move. This is because the process of obtaining marbled meat requires that the animal does not move and remains as fat as possible. They do, however, get massages here and there to ensure that they do not die prior to being used for the purpose of our oral pleasure.

So, we can acknowledge that movement is very important when it comes to health. As a matter of fact, I could quote dozens of studies that confirm that exercise improves our happy hormones and makes us feel less depressed.[128]

As we know, an animal that is not able to roam and move is not going to be a depression-free or stress-relieved animal, and, as a result, it is going to have high levels of stress hormones. When we eat this animal, where are all the stress hormones going?

So, we get it – movement is important. Why do Muslims 'move' five times a day? Before we get there, let us first speak about our physical cleansing process and how this ablution ties in with preventing illness and disease. In the absence of water, this can be performed with soil, but, for now, let us focus on performing it with water. Basically, we wash multiple parts of our bodies three times, including our faces, arms until wrists, mouth and nose, forehead, ears, and feet. We are also washing our hands, and we all know the benefits of having our hands washed and the importance of hand washing in the literature.

Let us move on to why we wash our mouths. The mouth can have food remnants left in there that will continue to feed pathogenic microbial growth unless we rinse it out, which we are doing one to five times per day prior to each prayer. So, in essence, we are preventing disease of the mouth, which affects diseases of the whole body, just by rinsing our mouths out.

Then we rinse our nose. As we breath from our nose, and as breathing from the nose releases a lot of N_2O (nitric oxide), which is a potent antioxidant, we are ensuring that any gunk stuck on the internal surface of the nasal passage is washed off so there is enough space for air to get through. We are also preventing disease here by physically removing particles that could otherwise make their way onto the tonsils, adenoids, and as far in as the lungs.

Just by the very mention of the few areas we are washing, we have a great understanding of how this physical purification is also, by nature, a measure to prevent sickness and disease.

On top of all this, there are acupressure points on the face that help with nervous tension and help calm the body. By the very act of washing our faces, we are turning on these pressure points and bringing our bodies to a state of calm.

In a nutshell, the craniofacial regions, which are very similar to regions washed or wetted with ablution, are important in brain cooling. So, when we wash our faces and the oral and nasal cavities, and when we wet the skull, we are helping the brain remain cool throughout the day.

When someone is in an erect position, the cerebrospinal fluid cannot optimally cool the basal parts of the brain. Of course, subhanallah, God is wise in relation to this because when a person is bowing or prostrating, spinal fluid is able to better flow between the brain and the skull.

During prayer, when we are bowing or prostrate, we are also maintaining or restoring the electrical contact between the human body and the earth. In yoga, the child's pose acts in a similar fashion. When we are praying on soil or another natural surface, or performing ablution alone, we are activating the parasympathetic nervous system, which regulates the movement of cerebrospinal fluid and purifies the body, therefore, reducing the risk of getting sick. As mentioned, the hygiene that comes with ablution also contributes to this.

Let us move on to active prayer and the science behind it. What is prayer? Prayer, or *salah*, is the spiritual practice performed by Muslims five different times throughout the day. While the spiritual significance is often discussed, the physical significance is sometimes overlooked. Therefore, I want to articulate how prayer promotes physical health and what is happening in the body as we move into different positions.

Prayer comprises a series of repetitive movements called *rakat*. Any Muslim who performs even just the compulsory prayer alone will repeat each unit of movements 17 times per day. One of the benefits of prayer is energy expenditure. These days, we live such sedentary lives; however, during prayer, we burn off excess energy, which can help prevent weight gain.

The interesting thing about prayer is that whatever is performed by the left-hand side is also performed by the right. For example, there is a standing position where the Muslim holds the left hand behind the left ear and the right hand behind the right ear, interestingly, hitting those acupressure points that control the parasympathetic nervous system. We perform the action with both sides of the body to activate both the left and right hemispheres of the brain. So, we are activating the spiritual or emotional centres of the brain but also the logical centres.

Vibration is the Essence of Life

In prayer, the way we breathe is also important. Breath control depends on which prayer is being recited. When we recite certain Arabic prayers, there are areas where we hold our breath and areas where we elongate what we are saying. As a result, we are activating the vagus nerve and causing a vibrational shift in our cells.

The Qur'an is super powerful because the frequencies of recited prayers reach the ear, move through to the brain, and affect cells through electric fields. Cells respond to these fields and modify their vibration. As Nikola Tesla says, energy, frequency, and vibration comprise the essence of the Universe.

So, in relation to the universe around us, we have proven that every single atom vibrates to a specific frequency. It does not matter if those atoms are a part of water, wood, or stone – everything in the Universe is vibrating.

Cells are the basic building blocks of our bodies. Each cell is made up of trillions of atoms, and each atom is made up of a positive nucleus with negative electrons rotating around it. Because of this rotation, an electromagnetic field is generated.

From a scientific perspective, when we recite the Qur'an, we cause the cells to vibrate at different frequencies, and each one of those frequencies has the ability to regulate and heal any health challenges, or any challenges in general, we are experiencing.

A French doctor by the name of Alfred Tomatis discovered that, of the human senses, our sense of hearing is one of the most important. He found that this sense controls the whole body and regulates vital operations, like balance and coordination.[129] We know this to be true because when we have, let's say, a middle ear infection, it can affect our balance and ability to walk. Further, the hearing nerves connect to the brain and, therefore, all other parts of the body, which explains why sound frequency affects the body as a whole. This also gives us a scientific basis for and understanding of a statement by the Prophet Muhammad (PBUH) that the Qur'an is the cure for everything except death.

It was not until fairly recently that we discovered that each part of the body has its own vibrational system, so each organ or group of organs that work in synergy with one another actually has its own vibration.

When we consider the whole picture and understand the absolute physical and spiritual benefits of prayer, we understand why the Islamic jurisprudence of missing prayer and having to make it up is as strict as it is. God has designed prayer to have immense benefits for us, while we consciously serve him in this three-dimensional realm.

Healing Power of Prayer

If we further elaborate, we can also find the importance of movement through prayer in somatic therapy. I have spoken about trauma and mental health and how it all ties into our spiritual and physical bodies in thorough detail to ensure that you really understand the importance of holistically analysing your health, rather than tuning out the symptoms. Somatic therapy is, in essence, body-oriented trauma therapy, where healing occurs through movement, which unleashes tension held in particular organs and parts of the body.[130] This relates to the trauma associated with the subconscious mind, where there is no present memory, no consciousness of what has happened. Therefore, nothing can be done because, quite frankly, there is no awareness of it even being there. So, while we pray and through prayer conduct particular movements, similar to somatic therapy, we encourage the release of tension and emotions stored in bodily organs that would otherwise continue to weigh us down. Through prayer, we are healing intergenerational and subconscious trauma. We are unconsciously healing from trauma that we have no conscious connection to.

So, God in His endless mercy allows us, through prayer, to heal from intergenerational trauma that not only did we not contribute to, but we had no consciousness of it being there in the first place.

We pray five times a day for many other reasons too. Primarily, we are keeping our physical connection with God. We are going to the prayer mat physically purified to realign, to recalibrate. When we are connected to a higher being, our chances of becoming hopeless, depressed, uncertain, anxious are low because this connection strengthens our knowledge around what we have control over and what we do not have control over. It allows us to remember and centre our lives around God, not the other way around. In doing this, it also helps us understand that this life is a temporary illusion, something that will come to an end, which means the pain and suffering we are feeling now are also promised to come to an end.

Prayer through recitation of particular surahs in the Qur'an are very healing in and of themselves. There are, for example, verses, such as surah Duha, that were revealed to Prophet Muhammad (PBUH) during his time of complete grief and sadness. This surah was revealed to him after a long period of no revelation. As he was not yet accustomed to bearing the weight of the revelation, he began to doubt himself and possibly assumed that Allah had forgotten him or was displeased with him. That is when surah Duha was revealed (Qur'an 93:1-11):

> By the morning sunlight,
> And [by] the night when it covers with darkness,
> Your Lord [O Prophet] has not abandoned you, nor has He become hateful [of you].
> And the next life is certainly far better for you than this one.

And your Lord will give you, and you will be satisfied.

Did He not find you as an orphan then sheltered you?

And He found you lost and guided [you],

And He found you poor and made [you] self-sufficient.

So as for the orphan, do not oppress [him].

And as for the beggar, do not repel [him].

And proclaim the blessings of your Lord.

If you were to analyse each sentence, you could certainly summarise the passage as one that tells man to be patient and that we are not alone, even in the times when we feel the most helpless and lonely. It moves on to mention that life is temporary, therefore, so are its challenges. It explains that we should not attach too much weight to our calamities and the hereafter is far more blessed and better for us, helping us have an objective perspective on our experiences in this realm. Then he promises that there are unimaginable rewards to come for those who are patient. He reminds us that he is the one, if he wills it, who will take us from darkness and place us into light. Lastly, it mentions the importance of remembering the less fortunate, being grateful, and ensuring the bond between us and God continues to be strengthened through perseverance and hope.

So, anyone who reads the English translation will feel like they just received the best pep talk ever to pull them out of their darkness.

Now, when we look at it in a different light, when we look at it in the light of pronunciation, we see even more benefits. This verse, similar to others, has something the Qur'an labels the 'qalqalah letters', which is a group of letters that makes an echoing sound, including daal, jeem, baa, tah, and qaaf. When you pronounce them, you are activating your vagus nerve. The vagus nerve is the longest cranial nerve in the human body, connecting to many internal organs, including our digestive organs, where nutrients are absorbed, assimilated, and transported to where they need to go. It helps regulate our heart, our breathing, and, thus, our ability to be grounded, our ability to stay in our parasympathetic nervous response, which is our 'rest and digest' response. In this state, healing takes place. The opposite to this is our sympathetic nervous response, which is our fight or flight mode, where we are in a state of stress and hyperactivity. The vagus nerve also forms a link between the gut and the brain. Scientists call this the gut brain axis, and it has the potential to reduce symptoms of depression, anxiety, and more.[131]

So, just in the pronunciation – the correct pronunciation in the Arabic language – we are activating the vagus nerve and, therefore, activating our parasympathetic nervous system, where healing takes place. Is that not beyond marvellous?

Let us now come to tasbih, a string of beads that helps us say certain Islamic words or affirmations a certain number of times. Many Muslims go about their days doing all of this, saying 'subhanallah' (glory be to God) 33 times, and 'alhamdulillah' (gratitude to Allah) 33 times, and 'allahu akbar' (God is great) 33 times and never question why there is a number attached. Why is it not ten times? Why not once? Through quantum physics, we understand the importance of how saying certain things a certain number of times has the ability to change the vibration of cells, causing healing to take place. Through the very movement of cells, aka cellular oscillation, the body cleanses and heals itself.

Traditionally, there was no apparatus used. Instead, we would use each bend of our finger to represent the affirmation once. Later, the tasbih, a string with 33 or 99 beads to help with the count and also to help with grounding, was invented. Because the apparatus is generally made from a tree or something of nature, such as ceramic or glass, it has the ability to ground the human body.

When you look at scientific literature around the benefits of grounding – aka exposing a part of your body, such as your feet, to the soil, where the negative ions or the free radicals are then transferred to the ground via the pull of the positive ions and minerals in the soil – it is similar to what is happening when we say a particular affirmation.[132] We are activating the vagus nerve and then holding on to a substance from the Earth to discharge any negative ions that are in the body. This is why prayer is a gateway to healing not only our spiritual bodies but our physical bodies too.

WHAT WE HAVE LEARNED ON OUR JOURNEY TOGETHER

It has taken me many pages to explain the connection between God and man, and the connection between man and himself, with his spiritual body, his physical body, and his connection to everything around him. I have spoken about acknowledging every single contributing factor to a particular symptom or a disease as being the foundational factor to healing. I have spoken about the importance of understanding why we behave in particular ways when it comes to food, why we overeat, overdrink, oversleep. We now know that understanding why we do certain things is the only authentic path to healing that behaviour.

We have spent many pages speaking on the science behind animal slaughter and the concept of man being the vicegerent of all beings. We delved into the ethics of life, something most of us are so disconnected from. Where does our food come from? How did it get here? Was it fair? Was it just? Was it sustainable? Why does any of this matter?

I have taken you on a journey of reflection, re-enactment, down memory lane, a journey of my highs and lows, my own shortcomings, my victories, and my continued desire to do everything within my power to share my experiences and knowledge. My goal is not to change anyone's mind or persuade them – that is not the business I am in. Instead, I aim to share my understanding of how this puzzle called health and life connects on realms that are conscious to us, and those that are uncon-scious to us, so perhaps my weeping soul can gain some remuneration in the hereafter.

There is so much unlearning to do, isn't there? So much of what you thought was the gospel actually fell short. So much of what you thought was history was actually his-story. Nothing is more painful but equally liberating than the opportunity to connect with the truth, within and outside of yourself. That is what life has taught me.

There were many times when I wished to blame others when, in fact, to regain my power and liberty, I had to first identify the shadows and unhealed parts of my very own being. Finally, I understood that the handcuffs of self-pity and the behaviours that disconnected me from the divine kept me locked up in a superficial world, void of happiness. I pray from the depths of my heart, where my shadows used to hide, that you benefit in more ways than you could ever fathom from reading this book. I pray that God blessed you to have the ability to turn the knowledge into action.

So, let us continue to read… Iqra bismirabbekellethee khalak. qalakal insane meen alak. Read, in the name of your lord, who created man from a clinging clot.

ACKNOWLEDGEMENTS

I would like to thank my mother, my mother, my mother, and then my father.

My mother is the reason why I am who I am and where I am today. My mother, who pushed me to my limits, even when I thought I had nothing else left in me. Who taught me my strengths, who taught me kindness and compassion. My mother, who taught me to never settle for anything less than what I deserve. My mother, who taught me to take up space in this world, to see myself before anyone else did. My mother, who saw my potential before I ever did. I love you, Mum, and words will never be enough to show my gratitude to you.

My father. The comfort your smile would give me when you would come home after your 14-hour daily taxi shifts. The sense of safety I would feel when you got home and I hugged you and breathed in your scent, which I would try and sniff out throughout the day when I felt anxious or stressed. You taught me, Baba, to be happy with whatever Allah had decreed. Never had I heard a word of complaint come out of your mouth after hours of driving a cab around Melbourne. Baba, I could never in a million years give you back even an ounce of what you have given me. May Allah forever bless you in this life and the one to come.

To my husband. Thank you for always being by my side, for supporting me, sometimes being my shoulder to cry on, other times my torchbearer. You will always be my 6'4" teddy. Thank you for loving me as I am. Thank you for loving the parts of me I never knew how to love myself. I love you.

My Elisa. You taught me unconditional love like no other, annem. Thank you for showing me all of the unhealed parts in me and thank you for patiently persevering on this journey with me, for holding space for me. Your smile will always melt my heart.

Alparslan, I pray one day you will read this book as a young man and acknowledge how much of my love for you went into it. My second born, you continued to hold the torch for mummy to see into her wounds; you helped Mum heal. You are everything I have ever wanted.

Elanur, my heart. I continued to write this book while you grew inside of me. Then you came earthside, and I felt a connection with Allah through your labour that I had never felt before. You are beautiful; you are fierce. You are not short of a dream come true.

To everyone else who showered me with love, who shook me at my core, who showed me my shadows, who triggered me, who gave me an opportunity to turn within, who shattered me, who broke me down, and who allowed for the light to enter. My friends, my clients, my extended family, and everyone else who has inspired the story of this life. I will forever be grateful for and humbled by the lessons and the blessings.

ABOUT THE AUTHOR

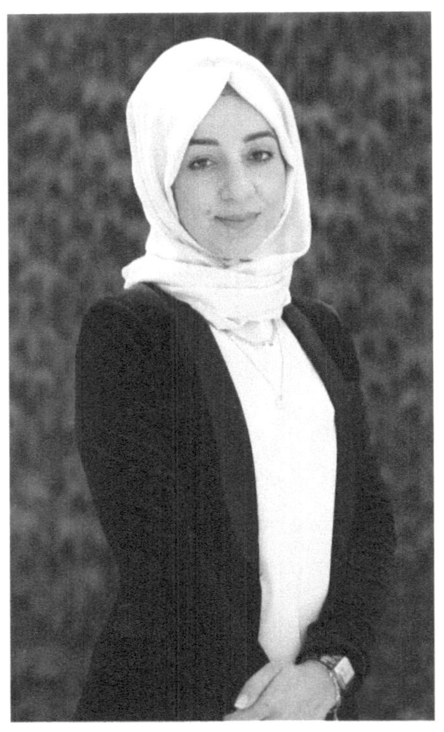

Julide Turker is a functional medicine practitioner with over a decade of experience. She helps people with health challenges by establishing healthy protocols unique to them and their situations. Julide facilitates healing by making changes to people's diets, lifestyles, and through supplementation with herbs and nutritional medicine. In short, natural medicine is a person-centred rather than symptom-centred approach.

Julide holds a bachelor of health science (naturopathy and nutrition) and a master of food sciences/food engineering from Melbourne University. She is also a personal trainer and neurolinguistic programming (NLP) coach.

Since 2022, Julide has focused on paediatric naturopathy. That is, she works with children under the age of 12. Her work is built on the fundamentals of Islam and the belief that our bodies are an amanah (trust) from Allah (God) SWT. She is committed to helping her paediatric patients restore their health and enabling them to be the best versions of themselves spiritually, physically, and mentally.

Julide is a mother of three angels and has been working from home via Zoom and phone consultations since the birth of her first child, during which time her clinic has grown rapidly, as individuals globally seek her out to support and restore their children's health.

In her free time, she enjoys reading, painting, and gardening, and she loves Beethoven, world history, literature, and the liberal arts. She is also a black belt dan one in taekwondo.

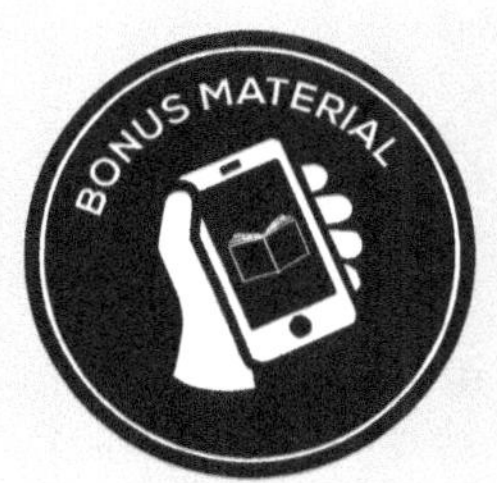

Julide is sharing more
in her BONUS CONTENT.

Scan the QR code or visit
www.julideturkernw.com/product/
one-third-of-your-stomach/bonus-content
to access additional content.

ENDNOTES

1   An-Nawawi 34.

2   Ryckmans, J n.d., *Arabian Religion*, online article, Britannica, viewed 21 January 2023, https://www.britannica.com/topic/Arabian-religion.

3   Ullmann, M 1997, *Islamic Medicine*, Edinburgh University Press, Edinburgh, p 1.

4   Ullmann, M 1997, *Islamic Medicine*, Edinburgh University Press, Edinburgh, p 1.

5   Ullmann, M 1997, *Islamic Medicine*, Edinburgh University Press, Edinburgh, p 3.

6   Tasgheer, A & Ishfaq M 2021, 'Female Infanticide in Pre-Islamic Arab Society: A Quranic and Historical Perspective', *Al-Qawārīr*, vol 3, no 1, viewed 6 July 2022, http://journal.al-qawarir.com/index.php/alqawarir/article/view/128.

7   Mirza Ghulam Ahmad, H 2008, *Ruhani Khaza'in*, vol 9, p 352.

8   Holm, DA, Ochsenwald, WL & Owen, L n.d., *Climate of the Arabian Desert*, online article, viewed 21 January 2023, https://www.britannica.com/place/Arabian-Desert/Climate.

9   van Beek, GW 1958, 'Frankincense and Myrrh in Ancient South Arabia', *Journal of the American Oriental Society*, vol 78, no 3, p 142, viewed 6 July 2022, https://doi.org/10.2307/595284.

10 Al-Yasiry, AR, Kiczorowska, B 2016, 'Frankincense – Therapeutic Properties', *Postepy Hig Med Dosw (Online)*, vol 4, no 70, pp 380-391, viewed 5 July 2023, doi:10.5604/17322693.1200553.

11 Han, X, Rodriguez, D & Parker, TL 2017, 'Biological Activities of Frankincense Essential Oil in Human Dermal Fibroblasts', *Biochimie Open*, pp 31-35, viewed 6 July 2022, https://doi.org/10.1016/j.biopen.2017.01.003.

12 Sunan Ibn Majah 3349.

13 World Health Organization 2020, *The Top 10 Causes of Death*, WHO, viewed 21 January 2023, https://www.who.int/news-room/fact-sheets/detail/the-top-10-causes-of-death.

14 Linhart, C et al. 2017, 'Use of Underarm Cosmetic Products in Relation to Risk of Breast Cancer: A Case-Control Study', *EBioMedicine*, vol 21, pp 79-85, viewed 21 January 2023, https://doi.org/10.1016/j.ebiom.2017.06.005; Darbre, PD 2005, 'Aluminium, Antiperspirants and Breast Cancer', *Journal of Inorganic Biochemistry*, vol 99, no 9, pp 1912-9, viewed 21 January 2023, https://doi.org/10.1016/j.jinorgbio.2005.06.001.

15 Arshad, H, Mehmood, MZ, Shah, MH & Abbasi, AM 2020, 'Evaluation of Heavy Metals in Cosmetic Products and Their Health Risk Assessment', *Saudi Pharmaceutical Journal*, vol 28, no 7, pp 779-790, viewed 21 January 2023, https://doi.org/10.1016/j.jsps.2020.05.006.

16 Brand, RA 2009, 'Biographical Sketch: Otto Heinrich Warburg, PhD, MD', *Clinical Orthopaedics and Related Research*, vol 468, no 11, pp 2831-2832, viewed 21 January 2023, https://doi.org/10.1007/s11999-010-1533-z.

17 Moen, I & Stuhr, LEB 2012, 'Hyperbaric Oxygen Therapy and Cancer – a Review', *Targeted Oncology*, vol 7, no 4, pp 233-242, viewed 21 January 2023, https://doi.org/10.1007/s11523-012-0233-x.

18 Hopkins, E, Sanvictores, T & Sharma, S 2022, 'Physiology, Acid Base Balance', *StatPearls*, viewed 21 January 2023, https://www.ncbi.nlm.nih.gov/books/NBK507807/.

19 Liberti, MV & Locasale, JW 2016, 'The Warburg Effect: How Does it Benefit Cancer Cells?', *Trends in Biochemical Sciences*, vol 41, no 3, pp 211-218, viewed 22 January 2023, https://doi.org/10.1016/j.tibs.2015.12.001.

20 Sender, R, Fuchs, S & Milo, R 2016, 'Revised Estimates for the Number of Human and Bacteria Cells in the Body', *PLOS Biology*, vol 14, no 8, viewed 21 January 2023, https://doi.org/10.1371/journal.pbio.1002533.

21 Xu, H et al. 2019, 'The Dynamic Interplay between the Gut Microbiota and Autoimmune Diseases', *Journal of Immunology Research*, vol 2019, viewed 21 January 2023, https://doi.org/10.1155/2019/7546047.

22 Cukrowska, B et al. 2021, 'The Effectiveness of Probiotic *Lactobacillus rhamnosus* and *Lactobacillus casei* Strains in Children with Atopic Dermatitis and Cow's Milk Protein Allergy: A Multicenter, Randomized, Double Blind, Placebo Controlled Study', *Nutrients*, vol 13, no 4, viewed 22 January 2023, http://doi.org/10.3390/nu13041169.

23 Wu, HJ & Wu, E 2012, 'The Role of Gut Microbiota in Immune Homeostasis and Autoimmunity', *Gut Microbes*, vol 3, no 1, pp 4-14, viewed 21 January 2023, https://doi.org/10.4161/gmic.19320.

24 Strzepa, A et al. 2018, 'Antibiotics and Autoimmune and Allergy Diseases: Causative Factor or Treatment?', *International Immunopharmacology*, vol 65, pp 328-341, viewed 21 January 2023, https://doi.org/10.1016/j.intimp.2018.10.021.

25 Langdon, A, Crook, N & Dantas, G 2016, 'The Effects of Antibiotics on the Microbiome Throughout Development and Alternative Approaches for Therapeutic Modulation', *Genome Medicine*, vol 8, no 39, viewed 21 January 2023, https://doi.org/10.1186/s13073-016-0294-z.

26 Jacoby, GA & Low, KB 1980, 'Appendix C, Genetics of Antimicrobial Resistance', *The Effects on Human Health of Subtherapeutic Use of Antimicrobials in Animal Feeds*, National Academies Press, USA.

27 Munita, JM & Arias, CA 2016, 'Mechanisms of Antibiotic Resistance', *Microbiology Spectrum*, vol 4, no 2, viewed 22 January 2023, https://doi.org/10.1128/microbiolspec.VMBF-0016-2015.

28 Drummond, RA et al. 2022, 'Long-term Antibiotic Exposure Promotes Mortality after Systemic Fungal Infection by Driving Lymphocyte Dysfunction and Systemic Escape of Commensal Bacteria', *Cell Host & Microbe*, vol 30, no 7, pp 1020-1033, viewed 5 July 2023, https://doi.org/10.1016/j.chom.2022.04.013.

29 Barrett, B 2018, 'Viral Upper Respiratory Infection', *Integrative Medicine*, pp 170–179, viewed 22 January 2023, https://doi.org/10.1016/B978-0-323-35868-2.00018-9.

30 Zhao, Y et al. 2009, 'Linkage Disequilibrium between Two High-Frequency Deletion Polymorphisms: Implications for Association Studies Involving the *glutathione-S transferase* (*GST*) Genes', *PLOS Genetics*, vol 5, no 5, viewed 23 January 2023, https://doi.org/10.1371/journal.pgen.1000472.

31 Madrigano, J et al. 2011, 'Prolonged Exposure to Particulate Pollution, Genes Associated with Glutathione Pathways, and DNA Methylation in a Cohort of Older Men', *Environmental Health Perspectives*, vol 119, no 7, pp 977-982, https://doi.org/10.1289/ehp.1002773.

32 McKay, DL et al. 2010, 'Chronic and Acute Effects of Walnuts on Antioxidant Capacity and Nutritional Status in Humans: A Randomized, Cross-Over Pilot Study', *Nutrition Journal*, vol 9, no 21, viewed 23 January 2023, https://doi.org/10.1186/1475-2891-9-21.

33 Crenshaw, BJ et al. 2018, 'Exosome Biogenesis and Biological Function in Response to Viral Infections', *The Open Virology Journal*, vol 12, pp 134-148, viewed 23 January 2023, https://doi.org/10.2174/1874357901812010134.

34 Hessvik, NP & Llorente, A 2018, 'Current Knowledge on Exosome Biogenesis and Release', *Cellular and Molecular Life Sciences*, vol 75, no 2, pp 193-208, viewed 21 January 2023, https://doi.org/10.1007/s00018-017-2595-9.

35 Lu, H & Mackie, K 2016, 'An Introduction to the Endogenous Cannabinoid System', *Biological Psychiatry*, vol 79, no 7, pp 516-525, 10.1016/j.biopsych.2015.07.028.

36 Manzanares, J, Julian, MD & Carrascosa, A 2006, 'Role of the Cannabinoid System in Pain Control and Therapeutic Implications for the Management of Acute and Chronic Pain Episodes', *Current Neuropharmacology*, vol 4, no 3, pp 239-257, viewed 21 January 2023, https://doi.org/10.2174/157015906778019527.

37 Goodfellow, CF et al. 1983, 'Oxytocin Deficiency at Delivery with Epidural Analgesia', *British Journal of Obstetrics and Gynaecology*, vol 90, no 3, pp 214–219, viewed 5 July 2023, https://doi.org/10.1111/j.1471-0528.1983.tb08611.x

38 Houlihan, J et al. 2005, *Body Burdens: The Pollution in Newborns*, online article, EWG, viewed 21 January 2023, https://www.ewg.org/research/body-burden-pollution-newborns.

39 Eidi, M et al. 2010, 'Seminal Plasma Levels of Copper and Its Relationship with Seminal Parameters', *Iranian Journal of Reproductive Medicine*, vol 8, no 2, pp 60-65, viewed 21 January 2023, https://www.researchgate.net/publication/45258378_Seminal_plasma_levels_of_copper_and_its_relationship_with_seminal_parameters.

40 Smith, JP 2009, 'Reconstructing Childhood Health Histories', *Demography*, vol 46, no 2, pp 387-403, viewed 23 January 2023, https://doi.org/10.1353/dem.0.0058.

41 Booth, FW, Chakravarthy, MV & Spangenburg, EE 2002, 'Exercise and Gene Expression: Physiological Regulation of the Human Genome through Physical Activity', *The Journal of Physiology*, vol 543 (pt 2), pp 399-411, viewed 5 July 2023, https://doi.org/10.1113/jphysiol.2002.019265.

42 Hodgins-Davis, A & Townsend, JP 2009, 'Evolving Gene Expression: from G to E to G×E', *Trends in Ecology & Evolution*, vol 24, no 12, pp 649-658, viewed 23 January 2023, https://doi.org/10.1016/j.tree.2009.06.011.

43 Zhang, L et al. 2019, 'Mechanism of Methylation and Acetylation of High *GDNF* Transcription in Glioma Cells: A Review', *Heliyon*, vol 5, no 6, viewed 24 January 2023, https://doi.org/10.1016/j.heliyon.2019.e01951.

44 Strandwitz, P 2018, 'Neurotransmitter Modulation by the Gut Microbiota', *Brain Research*, vol 1693, pp 128-133, viewed 24 January 2023, https://doi.org/10.1016/j.brainres.2018.03.015.

45 Schulte, EM, Avena, NM & Gearhardt, AN 2015, 'Which Foods May Be Addictive? The Roles of Processing, Fat Content, and Glycemic Load', *PLOS One*, vol 10, no 2, viewed 24 January 2023, https://10.1371/journal.pone.0117959.

46 Sahih al-Bukhari 287.

47 Imam Ibn Qayyim Al-Jauziyah 2010, *Healing with the Medicine of the Prophet*, Darussalam
    Publishers & Distributors, Saudi Arabia.

48 Al-Ghazali, AH 2016, *Al-Ghazali on Disciplining the Soul and on Breaking the Two Desires: Books XXII
    and XXIII of the Revival of the Religious Sciences (Ihya' 'Ulum al-Din)*, 2nd edn, The Islamic Texts
    Society.

49 Maté, G 2019, *Scattered Minds: The Origins and Healing of Attention Deficit Disorder*, Vermilion,
    London.

50 The Wisdom of Trauma n.d., *The Wisdom of Trauma*, webpage, Science and Nonduality, viewed
    24 January 2023, https://thewisdomoftrauma.com/.

51 Tongar, HK 2019, *Korkutarak Degil Sevdirerek Din Egitimi*.

52 Sahih al-Bukhari 6011.

53 Winfrey, O & Perry, B 2021, *What Happened to You?: Conversations on Trauma, Resilience, and Healing*,
    Flatiron Books, New York.

54 Maté, G 2021, *The Wisdom of Trauma*, documentary film, Science and Nonduality, https://
    thewisdomoftrauma.com/.

55 Van der Kolk, B 2014, *The Body Keeps the Score: Mind, Brain and Body in the Transformation of
    Trauma*, Penguin, London.

56 Hay, L 2014, *Loving Yourself to Great Health: Thoughts and Food – The Ultimate Diet*, Hay House,
    Carlsbad, California.

57 Al-Adab Al-Mufrad 1183.

58 de Weerth, C, Buitelaar, JK & Beijers, R 2013, 'Infant Cortisol and Behavioral Habituation
    to Weekly Maternal Separations: Links with Maternal Prenatal Cortisol and Psychosocial
    Stress', *Psychoneuroendocrinology*, vol 38, no 12, pp 2863-2874, viewed 5 July 2023, https://doi.
    org/10.1016/j.psyneuen.2013.07.014.

59 Maté, G 2019, *Scattered Minds: The Origins and Healing of Attention Deficit Disorder*, Vermilion,
    London.

60 Middlemiss, W et al. 2012, 'Asynchrony of Mother-Infant Hypothalamic-Pituitary-Adrenal
    Axis Activity Following Extinction of Infant Crying Responses Induced During the
    Transition to Sleep', *Early Human Development*, vol 88, no 4, pp 227-32, viewed 25 January
    2023, https://10.1016/j.earlhumdev.2011.08.010.

61 Australian Association for Infant Mental Health, *Controlled Crying*, online report, AAIMH,
    viewed 25 January 2023, https://www.aaimh.org.au/resources/position-statement
    s-and-guidelines/AAIMHI-Position-paper-1-Controlled-crying.pdf.

62 Kilner, JM & Lemon, RN 2013, 'What We Know Currently about Mirror Neurons', *Current
    Biology*, vol 23, no 23, viewed 28 January 2023, https://doi.org/10.1016/j.cub.2013.10.051.

63 Sahih al-Bukhari 5199.

64 Morey, JN et al. 2015, 'Current Directions in Stress and Human Immune Function', *Current
    Opinion in Psychology*, vol 5, pp 13-17, viewed 5 July 2023, https://doi.org/10.1016/j.
    copsyc.2015.03.007.

65 Sahih Muslim 45a.

66 Sunan al-Tirmidhi 2499.

67   Haneke, E 2015, 'Managing Complications of Fillers: Rare and Not-So-Rare', *Journal of Cutaneous and Aesthetic Surgery*, vol 8, no 4, pp 198-210, viewed 28 January 2023, https://doi.org/10.4103/0974-2077.172191.

68   Bridges, AJ 1995, 'Rheumatic Disorders in Patients with Silicone Implants: A Critical Review', *Journal of Biomaterials Science Polymer Edition*, vol 7, no 2, pp 147-157, viewed 28 January 2023, https://doi.org/10.1163/156856295x00661.

69   Whitslar, WH 1901, 'Dental Neurology', *The Dental Register*, vol 55, no 2, pp 55-71, viewed 2 February 2023, https://www.ncbi.nlm.nih.gov/pmc/articles/PMC6991328/pdf/dentreg135197-0001.pdf.

70   Qayyim, I 2015, *Provisions for the Hereafter*, Darussalam Publishers, Saudi Arabia.

71   Prentice, AM 2001, 'Overeating: The Health Risks', *Obesity Research*, vol 9, no 11, pp 234-238, viewed 2 February 2023, https://doi.org/10.1038/oby.2001.124.

72   Pi-Sunyer, X 2009, 'The Medical Risks of Obesity', *Postgraduate Medicine*, vol 121, no 6, pp 21-33, viewed 2 February 2023, https://doi.org/10.3810/pgm.2009.11.2074.

73   Quran Classes, *Eating Less: Science Validates Sunnah Yet Again*, online article, viewed 5 July 2023, http://quranclasses.net/eating-less-science-validates-sunnah-yet-again/.

74   Sunan Abi Dawud 2356.

75   Lahne, J 2019, 'Food Combinations and Food and Beverage Combinations in Meals', in HL Meiselman (ed), *Context*, Woodhead Publishing, Sawston, United Kingdom, pp 307-321.

76   All That Grows n.d., *GMO, Hybrid, Organic, and Heirloom Seeds. What's The Difference?*, online article, All That Grows, viewed 2 February 2023, https://www.allthatgrows.in/blogs/posts/gmo-hybrid-organic-heirloom-seeds-difference.

77   Omobowale, EB, Singer, PA & Daar, AS 2009, 'The Three Main Monotheistic Religions and GM Food Technology: An Overview of Perspectives', *BMC International Health and Human Rights*, vol 9, no 18, viewed 5 July 2023, https://doi.org/10.1186/1472-698X-9-18.

78   Johansson, I et al. 2010, 'Snacking Habits and Caries in Young Children,' *Caries Research*, vol 44, no 5, pp 421-30, viewed 3 February 2023, https://doi.org/10.1159/000318569.

79   O'Doherty, MG et al. 2011, 'Dietary Fat and Meat Intakes and Risk of Reflux Esophagitis, Barrett's Esophagus and Esophageal Adenocarcinoma', *International Journal of Cancer*, vol 129, no 6, pp 1493-502, viewed 3 February 2023, https://doi.org/10.1002/ijc.26108.

80   Food Standards Australia New Zealand 2007, *Consideration of Mandatory Fortification with Iodine for Australia and New Zealand*, report, viewed 3 February 2023, https://www.foodstandards.gov.au/code/proposals/documents/P1003%20SD11%20-%20Food%20Technology%20Report.pdf.

81   Ibn Qayyim al Jawziyya 2009, *The Prophetic Medicine*, Islamic Book Service.

82   DiNicolantonio, JJ & Berger, A 2016, 'Added Sugars Drive Nutrient and Energy Deficit in Obesity: A New Paradigm', *Open Heart*, vol 3, no 2, viewed 3 February 2023, https://doi.org/10.1136/openhrt-2016-000469.

83   Imam Ibn Qayyim Al-Jauziyah 2010, *Healing with the Medicine of the Prophet*, Darussalam Publishers & Distributors, Saudi Arabia.

84   Sunan Abi Dawud 3753.

85   Strandwitz, P 2018, 'Neurotransmitter Modulation by the Gut Microbiota', *Brain Research*, vol 1693, pp 128-133, https://doi.org/10.1016/j.brainres.2018.03.015.

86   Imam Ibn Qayyim Al-Jawziyya 1993, *Natural Healing with the Medicine of the Prophet (Tibbu-Nabawi)* (Al-Akili, M trans), Pearl Publishing House.

87   Sunan al-Tirmidhi 2380.

88   Hall, KD et al. 2019, 'Ultra-Processed Diets Cause Excess Calorie Intake and Weight Gain: An Inpatient Randomized Controlled Trial of *Ad Libitum* Food Intake', *Clinical and Translational Report*, vol 30, no 1, pp 67-77, viewed 3 February 2023, https://doi.org/10.1016/j.cmet.2019.05.008.

89   Niaz, K, Zaplatic, E & Spoor, J 2018, 'Extensive Use of Monosodium Glutamate: A Threat to Public Health?', *EXCLI Journal*, vol 17, pp 273-278, viewed 3 February 2023, http://doi.org/10 17179/excli2018-1092.

90   Sunan Ibn Majah 3355.

91   Kanz al-Ummal 3:460.

92   World Health Organisation (WHO), *World Obesity Day 2022 – Accelerating Action to Stop Obesity*, online article, viewed 5 July 2023, https://www.who.int/news/item/04-03-2022-world-obesity-day-2022-accelerating-action-to-stop-obesity.

93   Health Matters, *More Than 75% Of World Population Is 'Overfat': Study*, online article, NDTV, viewed 5 July 2023, https://sites.ndtv.com/healthmatters/75-world-population-overfat-study-343/.

94   Jami at-Tirmidhi 2380.

95   Emoto, M 2011, *The Hidden Messages in Water*, Atria Books, New York.

96   Colzato, L & Beste, C 2020, 'A Literature Review on the Neurophysiological Underpinnings and Cognitive Effects of Transcutaneous Vagus Nerve Stimulation: Challenges and Future Directions', *Journal of Neurophysiology*, vol 123, no 5, pp 1739-1755, viewed 16 May 2023, https://doi.org/10.1152/jn.00057.2020.

97   Elias, AA 2018, *Perils of Overeating in Islam*, blog, abuaminaelias.com, viewed 16 May 2023, https://www.abuaminaelias.com/the-perils-of-overeating-in-islam/.

98   Quran Academy 2017, *How the Food You Eat Affects Your Spirituality*, blog, viewed 16 May 2023, https://quranacademy.io/blog/how-the-food-you-eat-affects-your-spirituality/.

99   Animals Australia Team 2020, *How Are Animals Slaughtered in Australia?*, online article, Animals Australia, viewed 16 May 2023, https://www.animalsaustralia.org/features/how-are-animals-slaughtered-australia.php.

100   Carrasco-García, AA et al. 2020, 'Effect of Stress During Slaughter on Carcass Characteristics and Meat Quality in Tropical Beef Cattle', *Asian-Australasian Journal of Animal Sciences*, vol 33, no 10, pp 1656-1665, viewed 16 May 2023, doi:10.5713/ajas.19.0804.

101   RSPCA n.d., *Slaughter without Stunning*, webpage, viewed 16 May 2023, https://www.rspca.org.au/take-action/slaughter-without-stunning.

102   Australian National Imams Council (ANIC) 2023, *CAS Stunning Poultry Report*, report, viewed 16 May 2023, https://www.anic.org.au/wp-content/uploads/2023/05/ANIC-CAS-STUNNING-POULTRY-REPORT.pdf.

103   Bukhari.

104   Avena, N 2015, *Study Reveals That Cheese Triggers the Same Part of the Brain as Many Drugs*, online article, Mount Sinai, viewed 16 May 2023, https://www.mountsinai.org/about/newsroom/2015/study-reveals-that-cheese-triggers-the-same-part-of-the-brain-as-many-drugs.

105   Heart Foundation n.d. *Key Statistics: Cardiovascular Disease*, webpage, viewed 16 May 2023, https://www.heartfoundation.org.au/activities-finding-or-opinion/key-stats-cardiovascular-disease.

106   Terra Madre 2019, *What's the Difference between Organic and Australian Certified Organic?*, online article, viewed 16 May 2023, https://www.terramadre.com.au/information-centre/difference-between-organic-australian-certified-organic.

107   Terra Madre 2019, *What's the Difference between Organic and Australian Certified Organic?*, online article, viewed 16 May 2023, https://www.terramadre.com.au/information-centre/difference-between-organic-australian-certified-organic.

108   Department of Agriculture, Fisheries and Forestry n.d., *Organic and Biodynamic Produce*, webpage, Australian Government, Canberra, viewed 16 May 2023, https://www.agriculture.gov.au/ag-farm-food/food/organic-biodynamic.

109   Neeson, R 2010, *Organic Standards and Certification in Australia*, online article, Department of Primary Industries, viewed 16 May 2023, http://archive.dpi.nsw.gov.au/__data/assets/pdf_file/0011/353297/organic-standards-and-certification-in-Australia.pdf.

110   Department of Employment, Economic Development and Innovation 2009, *Artificial Breeding of Beef Cattle*, online guide, Queensland Government, viewed 16 May 2023, https://futurebeef.com.au/wp-content/uploads/Artificial_breeding_of_beef_cattle.pdf.

111   Agriculture Victoria n.d., *Code of Accepted Farming Practice for the Welfare of Cattle*, webpage, Victoria State Government, viewed 16 May 2023, https://agriculture.vic.gov.au/livestock-and-animals/animal-welfare-victoria/pocta-act-1986/victorian-codes-of-practice-for-animal-welfare/code-of-accepted-farming-practice-for-the-welfare-of-cattle.

112   World Health Organization (WHO) 2015, *Cancer: Carcinogenicity of the Consumption of Red Meat and Processed Meat*, Q&A webpage, viewed 16 May 2023, https://www.who.int/news-room/questions-and-answers/item/cancer-carcinogenicity-of-the-consumption-of-red-meat-and-processed-meat.

113   National Human Genome Research Institute 2023, *Carcinogen*, webpage, NIH, viewed 16 May 2023, https://www.genome.gov/genetics-glossary/Carcinogen.

114   The Guardian 2013, *How Much Water Is Needed to Produce Food and How Much Do We Waste?*, online article, viewed 16 May 2023, https://www.theguardian.com/news/datablog/2013/jan/10/how-much-water-food-production-waste; Ritchie, H, Rosado, P & Roser, M 2022, *Environmental Impacts of Food Production*, web page, Our World in Data, viewed 16 May 2023, https://ourworldindata.org/environmental-impacts-of-food.

115   Walder, F et al. 2022, 'Soil Microbiome Signatures Are Associated with Pesticide Residues in Arable Landscapes', *Soil Biology and Biochemistry*, vol 174, viewed 16 May 2023, https://doi.org/10.1016/j.soilbio.2022.108830.

116   Committee to Review the Health Effects in Vietnam Veterans of Exposure to Herbicides 1994, *Veterans of Agent Orange: Health Effects of Herbicides in Vietnam*, online book, National Academy Press, Washington, D.C., https://www.ncbi.nlm.nih.gov/books/NBK236356/pdf/Bookshelf_NBK236356.pdf.

117   Davoren, MJ & Schiestl RH 2018, 'Glyphosate-Based Herbicides and Cancer Risk: a Post-IARC Decision Review of Potential Mechanisms, Policy and Avenues of Research', *Carcinogenesis*, vol 39, no 10, pp 1207-1215, viewed 16 May 2023, doi:10.1093/carcin/bgy105.

118   Yan, H 2018, *Jurors Give $289 Million to Man They Say Got Cancer from Monsanto's Roundup Weedkiller*, online article, CNN, viewed 16 Mary 2023, https://edition.cnn.com/2018/08/10/health/monsanto-johnson-trial-verdict/index.html.

119   Jørgensen, PS et al. 2020, 'Coevolutionary Governance of Antibiotic and Pesticide Resistance', *Trends in Ecology & Evolution*, vol 35, no 6, pp 484-494, viewed 16 May 2023, https://doi.org/10.1016/j.tree.2020.01.011.

120   Morrison, HI et al. 1992, 'Herbicides and Cancer', *Journal of the National Cancer Institute*, vol 16, no 84, pp 1866-74, viewed 16 May 2023, 10.1093/jnci/84.24.1866.

121   Mannetje, A et al. 2005, 'Mortality in New Zealand Workers Exposed to Phenoxy Herbicides and Dioxins', *Occupational and Environmental Medicine*, vol 62, no 1, pp 34-40, viewed 16 May 2023, 10.1136/oem.2004.015776.

122   Sunan Ibn Majah 3266.

123   Sahih al-Bukhari 5376; Sunan Ibn Majah 3277.

124   Riyad as-Salihin 728.

125   Sunan Ibn Majah 3444.

126   Mitchell, SJ 2019, 'Daily Fasting Improves Health and Survival in Male Mice Independent of Diet Composition and Calories', *Cell Metabolism*, vol 29, no 1, pp 221-228, viewed 16 May 2023, https://doi.org/10.1016/j.cmet.2018.08.011.

127   Junnila, RK et al. 2013, 'The GH/IGF-1 Axis in Ageing and Longevity', *Nature Reviews Endocrinology*, vol 9, no 6, pp 366-376, viewed 16 May 2023, doi:10.1038/nrendo.2013.67.

128   Craft, LL & Perna, FM 2004, 'The Benefits of Exercise for the Clinically Depressed', *Primary Care Companion to the Journal of Clinical Psychiatry*, vol 6, no 3, pp 104-111, viewed 18 May 2023, doi:10.4088/pcc.v06n0301.

129   Tomatis Australia n.d., *What Is the Tomatis® Method?*, webpage, viewed 18 May 2023, https://tomatis.com.au/what-is-the-tomatis-method/.

130   Kuhfuß, M et al. 2021, 'Somatic Experiencing – Effectiveness and Key Factors of a Body-Oriented Trauma Therapy: A Scoping Literature Review', *European Journal of Psychotraumatology*, vol 12, no 1, viewed 30 May 2023, doi:10.1080/20008198.2021.1929023.

131   Kenny, EJ & Burdoni, B 2023, 'Neuroanatomy, Cranial Nerve 10 (Vagus Nerve)', *StatPearls*, viewed 30 May 2023, https://www.ncbi.nlm.nih.gov/books/NBK537171/.

132   Oschman, J, Chevalier, G & Brown, R 2015, 'The Effects of Grounding (Earthing) on Inflammation, the Immune Response, Wound Healing, and Prevention and Treatment of Chronic Inflammatory and Autoimmune Diseases', *Journal of Inflammation Research*, vol 8, pp 83-96 viewed 30 May 2023, doi:10.2147/JIR.S69656.